The Hidden Face of Pain

The Hidden Face of Pain

JACQUES SARANO
Translated by Dennis Pardee

JUDSON PRESS, Valley Forge

THE HIDDEN FACE OF PAIN

ISBN 0-8170-0469-6
Library of Congress Catalog Card No. 74-116726

Printed in the U.S.A.

Foreword

Jacques Sarano seeks to take the masks which pain wears from the face of pain and to introduce his reader to what pain in reality is. He disclaims any attempt to write a philosophical or biological study of pain, although I am confident that he does well in either field. His intention, instead, is "to slip his scalpel between the two" – biology and philosophy. He wrote a portion of the following pages when he was between the ages of twenty and thirty and the latter section on suffering as mediation between his thirtieth and his fortieth years. The book is written both from the point of view of a professional man, a medical doctor, and from the point of view of a personal witness to the meaning of suffering and pain *for him.* Sarano begins with the hypothesis that suffering is the *meaning* that we give to pain, the language and message that pain has for us. He continues with two "witnesses" to the meaning, the language, and the message that pain has for him as a person. Therefore, the book is *both* scientific and religious, an observation about the nature of pain by Sarano the scientist and a demand for the meaning of pain by Sarano the religious man.

Several motifs emerge within the pages of this book that have captured my imagination and made the book valuable to me. First, throughout the book, emphasis is laid upon the inseparable connection between meaningfulness of pain and bearability of pain. Sarano insists that the person whose pain has been explained to him is in a better condition to carry its weight than he was before this meaning was shown to him. Second, the *communal* nature of the meanings ascribed to pain is a persistent theme. As Sarano puts it, "I would believe less strongly in my own pain if no one else believed in it. . . . It is through other men that I grasp my suffering and theirs. . . . My pain inevitably includes what I have done with it for myself and others, i.e., how others have reacted to it for me." Therefore, in the third place, pain is an *incarnate* experience for both the individual and the community. Again, Sarano says that the soul that is incarnate is the only soul that suffers. Thus he emphasizes a distinctly Hebrew view of personality in his conception of both pain and the soul. In this connection, a whole section of the book is devoted to an explanation of the physiology of pain in terms that are easily grasped by the layman because of the relatively nontechnical discussion provided by Sarano. Finally, there is the theme of a unified view of pain set over against a separation of pain into normal and abnormal types of pain. Sarano says that such separations into different types of pain represent a philosophy in the guise of nomenclature. He rejects this classification and says that the true problem of pain is the *refusal* or lack of acceptance of pain in its disturbance of the total function of the person.

The mysterious function of the brain in producing consciousness presents man with his paradox of existence. The brain produces consciousness and thereby man is enabled to overcome his pain and at the same time is enabled to amplify his pain by his apprehension and memory. The brain "originates, orchestrates, and resists pain" at one and the same time.

In his personal testimony concerning pain and evil, Sarano points out that just because pain is insufficiently meaningful in the biological and scientific world is no justification for putting it to work for philosophy and religion. He speaks of pain as the problem child of science and the spoiled child of philosophy and religion. In turning to his second section on suffering as mediation, his personal testimony, he disavows any ambitions for a *summa theologica* in behalf of a personal testimony. Therefore, in this sense, the rest of the book is distinctly confessional in nature.

In essence, the second section of the book concentrates on evil, the hidden face of pain, which is a mediator between the self and the world, between man, the world, and God. He speaks of the muteness of pain in its naked versions and in its refusal to speak clearly of itself. He suggests that the muteness be given a "visa," that is, accepted as a stranger but welcomed even so. He insists that pain's refusal to speak may be the sufferer's ignorance of pain, his resignation, his retreat in the face of a scandal, his pride in having overcome difficulties, or his love afraid to make itself known. Sarano's confession is expressed succinctly in these words: "Evil is a reality only if I believe in God, if I love God and he loves me; otherwise, nothing would have any meaning; evil would reel along with the whole world." His concluding expression of his witness is in a theology of hope as the transcending power in the mysterious presence of God over the meaninglessness of pain. He says that the stranger in us speaks to the believer in us with the language of risk.

Sarano's testimony is clearest when he says: "We must learn how to look evil in the eye, just as it is, without being ashamed of it, or of God.

"And when we have observed the presence of evil, we have the right to refuse it, to combat it, to ignore it; it is perhaps more dignified to hold out our hand and go out to meet it. The loving attitude is better, not because evil is good in any way at all, but because it demands that we transcend ourselves, it requires *more* of us, more goodwill, more patience, more renouncement, more liberty."

I am personally intrigued by this contribution from this French physician. He is steeped in the existentialists' judgments about the absurdity of evil and uses the wisdom of Kierkegaard, Heidegger, Camus, and Sartre. He complements the findings of the American physician Harold Wolff on the subject of pain. I am "with" this author in his combined professional and personal approaches to the subject of pain. Frankly, I am assuming that probably this man had some "hand-to-hand combat" himself with pain between the time he wrote the first part of the book and the time that he wrote the second part. This personally oriented approach to the subject is, in my opinion, the only viable one because much pious drivel is written on the subject of pain by persons who have not known much pain, either of a physiological kind involving the central nervous system or of an interpersonal kind involving grief over significant loss, either by death, by divorce, by conflict with others, or over one's country's destiny.

The present book will be a vital contribution both to the meditative physician and to the minister who thinks below the surface of things. The interstimulation of thought between American pastoral care and the thinking of physicians and ministers on the Continent is intensified by this work. I commend it to the reader.

WAYNE E. OATES

Louisville, Kentucky

Contents

Part 1

*Pain, One Failure—
Master over Two Domains*

1

The Physiologist, the Physician, the Philosopher

"A defense reaction for the biologist, a source of moral uplifting for the philosopher, suffering for the physician, is only an evil he must combat." [1]

A good deal of this book was completed in the years 1957–1958. Then I abandoned it and have now taken it up again. Other concerns, medical and philosophical among them, interrupted its progress, but the basic idea was nevertheless reflected in a few articles and lectures.[2] I was struck by the strange paradox of pain appearing under two forms, with two faces: as both defense and trial — trial taking over after defense, or rather being absorbed in it, depending upon whether I adopted the logical or the historical order in working out an explanation. In either order, pain as defense and pain as trial are part of one problem.

In the formation of mentalities as in the psychology of an individual, pain as trial precedes pain as defense; it is an evil and a provocation for which someone must be blamed before its usefulness as a mechanism of biological origin can come to light. Only secondarily is pain's scientific status perceived, and that insight comes only by a war of attrition which shows itself slowly but surely to be of rational necessity. But at each stage of this conquest, domesticated pain, held in check under the guise of a vital defense mechanism, rebels against its limits, and primitive pain, untamed, reasserts itself in some unknown way when the first has lost its effect. Thus pain plays a double role, assuming a second mask when the first has failed: *one failure master over two domains* — this was too much for me.

[1] Paul Savy, *Traité de Thérapeutique Clinique* [Treatise in clinical therapeutics].

[2] Jacques Sarano, *Les Etudes philosophiques*, no. 4 (1959), *Présences*, no. 70 (1960).

So I did not intend to make a biological study of pain, nor a philosophical inquiry into suffering — I wanted to slip my scalpel into the joint between the two. How is the biologist to link hands with the sociologist, the scientist with the philosopher; how is defense pain to be linked with trial pain?

But when the two forms of pain were confronted, the real problem, lurking in the darkness of pain's ambiguity, shucked off its disguise and appeared as the real power behind the throne. For to express the contradiction inherent in pain and its double role is to declare that the *problem of evil* is no mirage but an ominous reality.

When the problem of evil reared its head, a second point of vital juncture (in reality but another form of the first) became apparent. The passage from defense pain to trial pain, from useful pain to problem pain, is the passage from the explanation of pain to its justification, the transformation from the scientific exploration of pain to a meditation on the philosophical and spiritual mystery of suffering.

This ancient problem of evil, which had obsessed me between the ages of twenty and thirty, has come back to the surface in another form; and the pages of a manuscript of that period have found their place in my present project which is the product of an entirely different outlook, so changed by experience and observation that I no longer recognize my former self. The present work follows the mainstream of my own evolution. It tells a story, the story of what suffering means to a man between thirty and forty.

Unequal in the Face of Suffering? Or Inequality of Suffering?

The history of a problem in an individual's life is but a part of the general human consciousness and its historical development. I have already stated that before appearing as an individual's response to life, suffering has already provoked a collective response from all of mankind. Its meaning for psychology and theology appears first: Suffering first of all appears as a part of a universal order; thus it becomes tolerable. And there is nothing less tolerable than an unexplainable suffering, one that is "simply too much." Its rationale must be greater than its cause — the anger of a god who must be appeased, a fault for which one must bear punishment.

Eliade has emphasized the coincidence in the aversion of primitive peoples for both suffering and any kind of *history:* Suffering is tied in with the perturbing and irreversible newness of the event. The primitive mind refuses the historical happening just as it refuses suffering. It neutralizes suffering by a double attitude of refusal: both toward individuality and toward history. Denying that either the individual or the event may be particular, primitive man eliminates time by means of rites for the cyclical regeneration of the world and by the repetition of archetypal gestures in which creation is born again, begun anew. Error, anger, pain — all are purified; time starts again at zero. Children are always glad to start over a game that was not going to their liking.

If only he had the time and the means, a physician would be capable of contributing his part to a psychological and sociological treatment of pain, to which one should really add a comparative work written from the same two standpoints. This book courts no ambition of that kind. Nevertheless, the very way in which different types of suffering have given body to my experience cannot have failed to leave its mark on my present project. More precisely, it has never ceased altering it, diverting it from its first line of progress, and I do not know if I must resist or yield to this warping. Now I neither see nor accept pain as I did ten years ago. The theoretical considerations of the problem have lost some of their meaning, and the language and manifestations of a mentality or civilization have received more of my attention.

When, for example, I hear my clients repeat, "I wouldn't mind dying, but I don't want to suffer," I cannot help leveling a slight criticism at their statement. In fact, I would be inclined not to accept them at face value and almost to reverse their terms. No, what is most frightening to *them* (and to *us*) is not the thought of suffering, but of dying. But Western man is so afraid of dying, and so afraid of suffering, that he no longer knows how to express what he fears most.

We could use the phrase "civilizations of suffering" to characterize Oriental man, who knows how to suffer and how to die. But the designation would better fit our own civilization where we know neither how to suffer nor how to die. We have progress — and we are retrograde. As Max Scheler has shown, the Greek-inspired civilization of the West has done its best to expel pain from its gates, and its progress is marked by the conquest of new zones of well-being and security from pain. This virile war is symbolized in the works of Hercules, and it is in very definite contrast with the Hindu concept of deliverance and also with Christian acceptance of suffering, but in a sense which we must yet state more precisely.

However, the progress of victory over pain has not been without retreats. While pain was withdrawing on one side, thanks to labor legislation and new techniques, it surfaced somewhere else, in haunts hitherto unknown or inaccessible, like guerilla fighters always able to replenish their forces. The comparison is incorrect; for pain is not something which takes up lodging in one place when removed from another. Rather, it identifies itself with our own response to an event; it flows with the blood in the healthiest veins of our overall personality. It is not on the order of an object, of what is possessed, but of the subject, of what *is*. This is why it is mockery to say of someone, "He has everything he needs to be happy." Quantitative or territorial gains in this area of human progress are won at the price of disadvantageous modifications which reduce our resistance to disease, exaggerate our sensitivity, our biological and psychological fragility toward pain. We may be better armed from a technical point of view, but we are morally weaker. The countries which we may call overprotected, or those individuals who have unlearned how to suffer, suffer more on the slightest occasion.

So when someone is concerned enough to ask that before anything else he be spared from pain, we must believe him. But no matter how cowardly he may show himself to be in the present trial, silent and prostrate or full of cries and groanings, this trial is nothing compared to the anguish felt as he discerns, or thinks he discerns, the obscure threats it holds for the future. The worst toothache, when it is understood and is clearly about to end, poisons the mind much less than the dull, suspicious pain in the depths of the abdomen for which the cause is unknown and the future unannounced. Man can tolerate a thousand times a disease which has been explained to him, but never can he endure an unnamed pain. He is afraid of dying, not of suffering.

Any victory of pain as a biological mechanism over pain as a trial of cosmic proportions must therefore appear in turn as a way of saving us from our weakness, a kind of exorcism – an exorcism which would fit in well with the methods of scientific objectivity. It is just as much an exorcism and a myth as Comte's evolution from the mythological to the positivistic age, from trial pain to useful pain.

We are living, then, in an age of uncertainty, in the ambivalence of pain's *double* function. It is on this problem that I have chosen to throw what light I have. All of us who have once suffered, who have seen others suffer, who have suffered from seeing others suffer

— ignorant and learned, well and ill, physicians and laboratory men, philosophers, believers and unbelievers — all of us, if questioned about pain, would surprise ourselves by giving, according to circumstances and persons, one or the other of these two profiles of pain, clearly delineated and, at first sight, difficult to reconcile. And the man who proffers one today will tomorrow resort to the other with no embarrassment.

Yes, it is possible for our age to furnish two *types* of explanations for pain: pain protects the living organism or is a result of the original sin, and it comes by the complicated avenues of the nervous system or by the no less complicated avenues of providence; pain is due to biological evolution or is a part of salvation. We explain pain in terms of the mechanism of pain or of its meaning.

This remarkable change of viewpoints is perhaps less indicative of the indecision and incoherency of us all than of the overlapping of two eras or of the duality of the creature itself.

When the hot stove burns us, it forces a cry from our lips, and our hand is immediately drawn back. I can understand this rapid warning which at the same time sets off the movement which saves my hand. I can even understand easily enough why the signal should be disagreeable, so evident is its usefulness. So we hardly ask ourselves any other questions, such as whether or not there are other means already at our disposal — quicker, surer, and painless. Is it better to learn by word or the example of our sense organs: "Don't go near the stove"; "Don't lean over the edge"? What painful warning mechanism could replace these means of avoiding the mortal danger of a fall or a wound?

Just as disconcerting and dumbfounding as some forms of pain are, so those of which I have just spoken are hardly bothersome and seem to leave us satisfied. I accept pain caused by a burn, a sting, a pinched finger, or a crushed thumb because I immediately see its origin. It is soothing to know who or what is guilty, and a confessed sin is already half forgiven. Moreover, the pain is followed so closely by its useful reaction that its undeniable necessity is demonstrated. A toothache or stomach cramps after a hearty meal may not be pleasant, but the pain enables me, forces me, to take the necessary measures of going to the dentist or of being on a diet for a day or two.

Such pain is a useful show of force and has a visible cause. (We even search out the cause when it is hardly evident. We have to find out why we have a sore back, and we give a cause such as, "I didn't cover myself well enough during the night — must have gotten cold.") These two assertions are favorable recommendations giving daily pain its license to practice. And pain's position as guardian of our body's well-being, of our complete health, loses no credibility.

Does this not make it all the more difficult to justify certain stubborn nervous diseases which slowly but surely destroy a life, but whose cause is unknown? (Whether the cause is unknown because of the sick person's ignorance or the doctor's, or because of the insufficiency of modern science is of no importance for our purpose here.) What they could possibly be a warning of is even more unknown. What are these diseases asking us to do; what do they want of us; what do they mean for us; and what are they trying to get us to do? Rest? Escape? Adopt a new life? We just do not know; we are helpless, nonplussed.

But how about the death of one's mate or one's children, the moral pain which we call grief and which is on an entirely different plane of experience? How is this pain to be explained as a defense mechanism? How are we to distinguish the exact point of juncture between pain, suffering, grief, anguish, anxiety, renal colic, and a toothache? Doubtlessly the simplest way would be to set aside several forms of pain, even to give them different names, and to reserve our term for the limited use of biologists and physicians. What is there in common between an individual's biological pain and historical catastrophes – wars, earthquakes, deportations? They both register hurt, of course – one on the doctor's scale and the other on the scale used by historians and prophets.

All of these forms of pain are in a sense identical, but also disproportionate. I touch the stove and burn my hand; I roll on the ground, contorted by a perforated ulcer; I die of cancer, wracked by waves of intolerable pain; I lose my child; my family is wiped out by an epidemic or an automobile accident; a flood in Hamburg counts its victims by the hundreds; a typhoon in Japan, a landslide in Peru, a volcanic eruption – each devastates a whole region, annihilates a continent. What unity may be seen in this graduation and discontinuity in the importance of different woes? What unity is there in the disproportion between a migraine headache and the Agadir earthquake, between yesterday's indigestion and the great woes of 1939–1945, or the wars in Algeria or in the Congo? What is the relationship between micro-pain and macro-pain, between the humble pain which the physician sees every day and that pain which reaches cosmic proportions?

The primitive mind makes the connection and considers his

suffering as homogeneous, or perhaps leaves pain in its original homogeneity. He is ignorant of purely biological pain and understands it psychologically as part of his cosmos. But we have discovered the "normal" pain described by the biologist. Is this discovery a part of man's evolution? Or have we found only a difference in proportions between two kinds of pain for which there is no common measure? Are there two kinds of pain, or two ways of looking at pain? Further on I shall deal more systematically with this problem on which the entire orientation of my study depends. But right now we can already see, in men's reactions to grief and affliction, two points of view which may already be observed in reactions to the slightest toothache. A person may accept the pain as normal for a decayed tooth, or he may ask, "What have I done to deserve such a thing?" These are two opposite attitudes in which the degree of one's common sense and one's philosophy of life become apparent. Depending on his attitude, the sufferer gets more, or less, profit from his experience than his neighbor who, at less cost, "puts himself in his place" and pities. Faith succeeds in ensuring a better recovery than skepticism, the strong man than the weak, the brave man than the cowardly, the wise man than the rebel. The diversity of pain seems to carry one over to the diversity of attitudes. Contradictory or complementary explanations and justifications are all, in reality, due to the well-known fact that men "are not equal in the face of pain" and just as much to the fact that pain itself is not equal. We can then understand what was at first astonishing, that pain is, at different times and for different people, a function in the service of life, a woe, a revolting nonsense, an evil — or, a reversal of the unjustifiable, a justifiable trial, liberating and life-giving.

Subjective and Objective Approaches to Pain

Pain is diverse, and men are diverse in the face of pain. It is a personal and an interpersonal experience. Its subjective aspects and objective data require the reconciliation of elements which are not always easy to bring together.

We must begin by admitting that there is, underlying every treatment of the subject, an intimate experience of pain which we could call naked pain. He who has not known and experienced naked pain in his body and in his heart has no way of knowing what we are talking about, except as a convention of speaking, as a man born blind might speak of colors.

There is no way of explaining this pain which must be lived

before it can be understood, experienced before it can be spoken of, except that it is less of a datum which precedes an alert consciousness than the very ground upon which our different experiences as adults rest. Naked pain is not to be grasped in itself, but it is present in all other forms of pain. All the others refer their origin to it. It is less of a limit than a point of reference. Although the civilized adult may occasionally offer it battle, how may we designate it, except as an immediate threat which anything living flees with all its might? *Courage* is one of man's spiritual energies most directly rooted in pain although the pain is no longer recognizable. Courage (which we might define prosaicly as a well-being obtained because an attempt has been made on my first well-being by an outside force) is made up of horizontal layers where not only physical and moral pain, the painful and the disagreeable, but also pain and exultation, extreme anguish and extreme joy alternate their influence.

Thus, all the most developed of man's inner experiences—courage, cowardice, cruelty, patience, and pity—all rest on the fundamental ground of naked, raw pain, uncategorized pain, which is in itself less an experience than the presupposition which *unifies* the diversity of painful experiences.

But can we speak of pain as being felt without the immediate support of an objective datum, a *language* of pain, a *form* of pain which must be described? Expression, behavior, and communication by word and by act furnish such essential information about a pain felt only within, so intimate that even the language of introspection cannot touch it. But we just said that nothing can be said about this raw pain except that it is presupposed as present whenever pain is mentioned.

The inner experience, which would appear to be the most concrete since its roots are sunk into the very heart of my existence, is in the end only an abstraction if it is not expressed in matter, if it does not take on the flesh and blood of a *body*. Physical or moral, a pain which exists necessarily becomes objective. Perhaps its progress is imperceptible, but its movement is nevertheless susceptible of being detected, measured, and recorded by an ideally precise instrument.

It would be incorrect to identify pain with a material phenomenon which could be physically recorded, for pain is a language and a message, the cry of suffering flesh and threatened life. However spontaneous it may be, this cry must be understood as an appeal. It is meant for someone. In the desert, the one who suffers is calling to someone — his mother or his God. His cry for help, his abortive attempt at communication, his decapitated hope for an answer, his invocation, his cry, and even the silence that follows, are all witnesses to the call for dialogue, for society, from the men and animals around us.

A completely silent pain is contrary to nature. I would even say that it is frightening. When distance within space or within the species keeps us from hearing cries of pain that we think should be coming forth, this absence of a cry appears to us as a robbed cry, a cry that has been kept back, gagged, or strangled. I remember having witnessed an undersea catastrophe. Its agony was deadened by a thickness of the water which stopped all communications. So it is with certain insects: Their mute suffering, deprived of either a look or a cry, touches us, if we deign to observe it, even more because it almost left us indifferent. We think the insect is speaking but that we cannot hear it or that something is keeping it from speaking.[3]

Yes, pain with no outlet by words, deprived of expression by word or act, is inhuman, contrary to nature. Would it still be meaningful as pain if beyond the absence of language its presence were still master — even though it were kept from speaking? Pain without a body is hardly conceivable. Only that soul which is incarnate can suffer.

There is an important corollary to this indispensable incarnation. I point it out now because it furnishes one of the principal themes of my study: Pain cannot be reduced to a pure suffering without taking on concrete form as an act. A movement, no matter how well hidden, even if it is only microscopically visible within the tissues, brings pain to the outside, but the movement is not purely an effect, a simple result (like one ball bumped by others), but an expression, a riposte, a language of revolt or appeal. Pain is therefore an indissoluble combination of suffering and acting, a passivity backed up by a reaction or way of behaving. It is both impression and expression, or, if one may say, inside and outside — in any case, an act.

The *objective approach* to pain thus obtains a supplementary legitimacy within its own life, as it were. This justification in no way reduces the difficulties, which we shall examine a bit later, of observation and experimentation with animals. For observable manifestations also have meaning, as part of a necessary circle, only

[3] I think also of the silence of Anderson's little siren or of the beast in the *Beauty and the Beast.*

by their constant reference to an intimate and unutterable experience of a subject's life. External manifestations are inseparable from internal experience and are nourished from that substance just as the sign is nourished by what it signifies. Unless our observations are rooted in life, we will be deceived by signs that lack this rooting.

Not without a *personal participation* do I witness behavior, gestures, and cries. I find them to be true and meaningful not because I reason by analogy, but because I share the experience directly, immediately, and sympathetically.

The comprehension of objective pain is an experience of shared subjectivity, an inter-subjective experience, we might say.

When I see a man or an animal suffering, I do not deduce that such is the case by deciphering the hieroglyphs of word or action. Rather, my experience spontaneously coincides with his; I live his suffering. Our pain for others, that of others for us, takes on such importance that if our individuality were reduced to its naked self, it would seem vain, with no consistency. The echo, the complicity, the confirmation of one person's suffering by another gives it a dimension that is beyond observable objectivity, but belongs rather to the inter-subjectivity of participation.

How many of the sick complain that they find no receptive echo in those around them and say: "No one takes me seriously!" "My husband can't understand that I am sick! He doesn't know what it is to suffer!" The most genuine pain, such as neuralgia, abdominal pain, or lumbar sciatica, still thirsts for consideration or, at least, for recognition. It doubts itself and becomes exasperated at being alone in its suffering. It no longer knows just what its own limits are; it lacks weight and measurements. I would believe less strongly in my own pain if no one else believed in it, or by reaction I would paint it larger than it is. For although I am near to my pain, I cannot put it to the test of truth. Am I imagining my illness? The scepticism that I feel in those around me makes me wary of myself.

In contrast with my lack of assurance as to my own pain, the sight of someone else's pain fills me with irresistible waves of sympathy. But analysis teaches me to be wary even here, for this knowledge by sympathy is direct. My brother's pain in which I imagined myself to be effectively participating, which I could feel, which I could touch, then dissimulates itself out of my reach.

My nerves are made for the currents of my own pain, not for those of someone else; neither are theirs made for mine. I alone know how I suffer.

But I can hardly grasp my own pain any more directly than that felt by someone else.

Man's inner sensitivity and his faculty of sympathetic participation have both come down through millenniums of civilizations and cultures. It is through other men that I grasp my suffering and theirs. Suffering is made accessible to me, and is separated from me, through the thick layers of my education, my own thinking, my false fronts, and my deepest moral, social, and religious convictions — my psychology, my character, my habits, and my attitudes.

In order for my pain to reach me (mine and anyone else's), it must traverse this immense culture. It is born and transformed in me by this culture.

Access to *my own pain* is through this intermediary and is refracted by language, by civilization, by conventions, stereotypes, and *signs*. Even so, my voyage into the sufferings of someone else is also by the intermediary of *analogous signs*. My knowledge is inexact, indirect, *symbolic,* as Caruso has said of all knowledge, of every encounter of man with his world. And my universe is just as foreign as that of anyone else.

Pain is a mixture of inner experience and outer manifestations. But it is impossible to experience a pain that exactly coincides with either the inner experience or the outer manifestation.

The reality of pain is never unmixed; pain reveals itself, then hides; is full of meaning but also of contradictions. It is always given to me by the means of its social signals, even when it is tearing me inside and out. Pain's reality is given to me imperfectly but genuinely by signs. Even when I am suffering the terrible destructiveness of a mortal attack, I cannot evaluate the depth of my pain. No one knows how much I am suffering. Neither do I.

There is no question of doubting my pain, as I may doubt yours. But how can I evaluate it? The question of suffering would be no less absurd even if its intensity could be measured. For every pain possesses an inimitable originality and qualities which cannot be measured. But there are varying degrees of pain, each more or less bearable, and this is what I am unable to evaluate alone. Let us say then that it is not my raw pain but my attitude toward (and with) it which is decided by my presence in society (should I consider it of some worth or scorn it?). But I contest that it is impossible to separate — although it may be easily distinguished — raw pain from my social attitude which is already an action.

As we draw it from our experience, still warm and alive, my pain inevitably includes *what I have done with it for myself and for others* — which may perhaps be stated as *how others have reacted to it for me.*[4]

Correctly speaking, there is no true, authentic pain — never gold coin, only bank notes.

Let us add that my own pain is, to a certain degree, seen from a distance, from outside, just as my view of someone else's pain is to a certain extent a view from within. There is no essential difference between the largely indirect perspective I have of my own pain and the perspective I have of another's pain in which I participate by a process of inner sympathy.

I am constantly making mistakes concerning pain which could leave the impression that it possesses a secret essence inaccessibly different from its appearance. However, pain *identifies itself with what it appears to be;* it is never anything other than what it gives itself to be through the signals our consciousness receives from it. Rather we should say that if pain is the sum of its disparate and conflicting appearances, this very conflict raises doubts in our minds as to its authenticity. Each detail is absolutely convincing; but when all are put together, their relativity makes them suspicious and redundant. If you want to discredit pain, just bring about a confrontation of differing witnesses. In order to have no doubts about my pain, I must be alone; but solitude rapidly becomes the surest way to doubt. The echo of my pain in others, their complicity in my pain, reduces it to a relative status just as surely as I needed them to assure me of my pain in the first place. Pain is confused with what it appears to be, but what is an appearance carried to the absolute degree except the opposite of absoluteness?

Whether or not I am mistaken concerning my present pain (the error here, as elsewhere, is only perceivable against the background of truth, whose presence provides the very possibility of error), it is always expressed by a half-truth. Whether or not I am mistaken concerning someone else's pain, my participation in it proves, not the objective quality, but the mixed character of the half-truth I am observing. For if the outer manifestations I am observing did not correspond directly with the inner experience, if it were not the lifeblood of the living pain, if this outer form were not a part and the very substance of *pain,* if the visible signs were but a translation of an inner foreign experience — how could I tremble, how

[4] A thought comes to my mind from an old book *La modestie de Dieu* [God's modesty]: "Pain is only poignant to the extent that it is barely visible. But it must at least be barely visible. Pain which did not make itself seen would be the most poignant if it were nevertheless perceivable." Pain is inseparable from what we call today being in the world, our relations with the world.

could I weep, how could I suffer along with my brother, how could I commune with what would only be a show? It is not enough to speak of a domino effect, with tears calling out tears, and these tears awakening emotion (as laughter provokes a good feeling, and adrenaline provokes anger after making one's hair stand on end). All this effect does is to give rise mechanically to a psychological or mixed psychological-social semblance of the original, an unnamed something which imitates the salty bitterness of my pain. "We can only imitate what we understand," Ruyer correctly writes. "We can only imitate the true meaning of something." Any imitation is due to at least a partial comprehension of the original, to a participation, a being joined to another; and it is not debasing it to give this comprehension the full weight of its corporeity, its flesh and blood.

For the body is what ties living beings together. The body divides, and the body unites. It is true that it isolates us from each other, but it is also what makes us husband and wife, sister and brother, in a solidarity which is strengthened by suffering as well as by joy. If souls were alone, they could not share their suffering; they could not suffer at all. It is said that the soul's transparency would bring down the barriers which divide us, but it would rather sterilize contact to such a degree that there would be no way of grasping our reality; all would be steep and smooth. But the barriers of the flesh constitute the cement which holds together the molecules of different pains, the rough cement whose very roughness makes the atoms of love stick together.

Pain on an Animal Level and Experimentation

To understand pain is to understand its corporeity, without which it could not even exist; to admit the necessity of the body; to admit that the objective approach reveals a meaning just as completely as the lived experience; and to grant this approach official rights, but not reserve for it any improper priority or dispense it from constant reference to the subject. It requires the acceptance of the idea of participation from an outside position, by the observation of behavior. I have no right to dig in behind the *secret* of my pain, pretending that I alone am able to say something about it. I can say something about the pain of others, as they can about mine.

Observation and experimentation carried out on an animal, even in a hermetically sealed environment, are nevertheless useful for understanding a real-life contact even though the conclusions to be reached are often implicit and quickly forgotten. Objectivity must be founded on inter-subjectivity.

Thus, subjectivity becomes abstract when it is cut off from its manifestations, its gestures. But neither must the objective approach be content with just these observed data: Sympathy, corresponding reactions, and analogies are equally deceiving and must be subjected to criticism. No partial datum can, without danger, take precedence over an all-inclusive experience — which is just the opposite of a datum.

One's language can precisely indicate pain and its many details, but language is often subject to exaggeration, superfluity, minimization, and deformation. Details are often added. I am always more or less mistaken concerning pain.[5] But how may I evaluate the situation *when pain includes this very deformation and is the sum of all that I feel and manifest, even my mistakes?* This is why asking if someone "is suffering less (or more)," or if he "is bearing his pain better," does not have much more meaning than (as I mentioned before) to say that a depressed person "has everything to make him happy." Any distinction between pain's "being" (an objective reality labeled *pain*) and its "appearance" is deceiving. Rather it is only an indication of our lack of comprehension toward others and of the separation between us. We shall see how improper and even scandalous it is to define, on the one hand, an objective reality and, on the other, a subjective experience, with the underlying assertion that there are pains "without an objective basis," just as some dare to assert that people "imagine" themselves to be sick.

I see a profound identity between "bearing," "overcoming," "knowing how to suffer," and "suffering less." At the best, a differentiation between these terms would be more or less consciously dependent on an ethical or social context, which has a direct effect on the quality of the pain itself (as Bergson has remarked concerning quantitative measurements of the intensity of an effort, a quality which must be understood as *sui generis*). Of course, indifference to woe, like insensibility to pain, must not be placed on a par with Buddhist or Stoic asceticism, nor cowardice with sensitiveness to evil (committed by or on the subject); the *road,* the secret of progress which leads to a quasi-absence or omnipresence of pain, must not be confused with the intensity of pain itself. In

[5] I am even incorrect in using the terms *more* or *less.* In this shady area of quantity/quality in which no measurements can be made, the intensity of pain is tied in with its *justification,* with what I know of its cause, with the importance that one may properly grant it. In short, its intensity is inseparable from its worth as a *sign.*

other words, our task is not to pass judgment on the objectivity of suffering, nor is it to try to discover if the pain is "deep-rooted" or not. Pain must be accepted at face value, for it is impossible to separate it from these very words and their snares.[6]

In any case, I am no less ignorant of the pain before me when I try to make myself a critic of it. My sympathy can only knock on this door as a blind man, with a groping touch. I can do my best to commune with someone's pain, but I never will know if the pain I feel for him is the same as his (neither will I ever know if my *red* and *bitter* are the same as his).

Language, faces, hands—openings and barriers to communication—and I come back to my preceding disclaimers: Pain is, in fact, a *secret*—mine or his—for me and for the other fellow. Any pain is a result, the end of a process; and no one can work back to it without critical analysis, a critical psychoanalysis and socio-analysis, endless and never accurate.

Perhaps we are now relatively certain to agree on the meaning of this word and the type of experience it represents. But what about our knowledge as concerns the pain of animals, higher mammals, or lower species? Most authors distinguish between an expressed behavior and a non-expressed behavior as a reaction to pain.

Perhaps pure and simple pain moves us more by its bewildering muteness, but should we be taken in by it? Helter-skelter flight; confused twisting and turning which often becomes harmful for the animal and even suicidal; a silent behavior but which includes all the symptoms of disorderly panic; "disastrous" behavior on the

[6] I cannot accept any distinction between experienced pain and "real pain" which is supposed to be the "normal" cause of the first, nor the logical conclusion that there is a hallucinatory pain which has nothing to do with "real" pain (cf. L. B. Geiger, *L'expérience du mal* [The experience of evil] in Casterman, *La souffrance valeur Chrétienne* [The Christian value of suffering], pp. 33 ff.). Pain cannot be compared with perception ("of something"): It is in itself its own proof. That is why it is just as revolting to say to someone in misery that he has "everything to make him happy." Moreover, this reference to what should "normally" hurt us, as any reference to what is "normal," is worthless. The death of my child is "normally" painful within a certain civilization or philosophy of life. In others (and they do exist) such is no longer the case, and there I would have "hallucinations" of evil! In pain as reality and as appearance, objectivity and subjectivity melt into the unity of an experience. Pain is an experience: Any "objectivity," "objective knowledge," or "reality" of pain is only a direct or indirect borrowing, admitted or secret, from an experience. Also, if it is true that the hurt we cause is not always felt, it is no less necessary to refer to an injury received in order to qualify as the one inflicted. The evil committed (a moral evil) must necessarily be stated in terms of the injury received. There is no precept which does not verify the law of reciprocity among men (for example: "Love your neighbor as yourself").

part of an animal, a plant, or an isolated cell — all these phenomena leave a considerable margin of error for our interpretations. We judge, we even feel with horror, that an earthworm cut in two is "writhing in pain," because we connect its agitation with the injury it has received and because its contortions resemble those of a man writhing in pain. But we have no way of knowing whether the worm may be really "feeling" a type of pleasure or nothing at all. However, in this case we do know. The example was poorly chosen: The caudal extremity is agitating because it has been deprived of nervous coordination, whereas the head is able to continue on its way. Chaotic behavior following an aggression, with an added superficial and sympathetic analogy to a human reaction, is enough to incite us to invent an inexistent pain and to delude ourselves as to its reality.

But *expressive behavior* seems to be of another nature, especially in the higher mammals (Buytendijk, however, studied it in the look of an octopus!). We no longer observe only a coordinated or uncoordinated defense reaction, but the intentional (in its objective sense) expression of suffering: cries or plaintive modulations of the voice, with a particular timbre, entirely different from sounds of joy, and a special look in the eye. But how many things are invented in a look! Such forms of expression almost make up a language. I mean to say that it is impossible to accept such an expression as purely and simply an effect caused by a disequilibrium, but that it must be a call, an intentional behavior.

Although it is difficult to mark out a tolerable limit for an interpretation by sympathy and also difficult to make a cut-and-dried distinction between an automatic behavior and expressive behavior (concerning neither of which can we say that it is a pure effect, nor can we deny that both have a certain meaning to them), it is, nevertheless, true that our approach to pain risks going over to the realm of fantasy as soon as we leave the most intelligent beasts if we admit that pain is a Janus-faced experience whose exterior form takes its meaning from within.

Our insistence on this point may be excused, in view of the data from medullary experiments practiced on animals from which *the brain has been removed* and on which some physiologists have set great store. I would in no way deny their usefulness in providing more exact knowledge as to the paths and centers of biological *defense*. But no matter how lively and useful defensive reaction to aggression may be (scratching, fleeing, kicking), defensive behavior is not pain, unless we transform our words and, even more, the basic meaning of the crucial experience which has provided the starting point and the center of reference for our study.

Here we are clashing with experimental science, and we must make ourselves clear. A dog with its brain removed responds to stimuli which are normally pain-inducing by crying, kicking, and running movements. Does this mean that it is suffering, that it feels pain? This is not our department, the physiologists answer; we define pain *objectively* as "sensitivity to pain-inducing stimuli," and this sensitiveness is understood in terms of behavior.

A distinction must be made, they add, between *pain* and consciousness of pain. Then they launch into a criticism of Lerich who dared to say, "There is no excitation which may be called painful as long as the brain has not had its say." Adding his voice to this criticism, A. Grasset,[7] for example, has gathered together several arguments based on experimental, surgical, and clinical findings with the purpose of proving that there is pain before or without the brain's function, before or without the complicity as it were of the psyche. Pain, the physiologists say, exists at the spinal stage and may be defined as "the combined spontaneous reactions provoked by a pain-inducing stimulus." Pain concerns the midbrain (mesencephalon) and the between brain (diencephalon) when the cortex or the pons has been removed from an animal's brain.

A prefrontal lobotomy performed on a human being also produces "experimental analgothymia."[8] The pain, we are told, has not disappeared, nor the knowledge of pain – what has disappeared is what we might call the painfulness of the pain. "After a lobotomy the person in pain is aware of his pain, but no longer does he suffer."[9]

But what is pain from which one does not suffer? Does it even merit the name of pain? Once it is reduced to a defensive behavior or to an indifferent "knowledge," it is no longer pain. When the person who has undergone a lobotomy tells me that he feels pain without suffering from it, I understand (if it is possible to *translate into words* the inexpressible feeling he has expressed) that he feels nothing painful *in what he and I both know to be painful.* The word "pain" has become conventional for him; he has kept the letter but lost the spirit. The word "pain" no longer has the meaning

[7] A. Grasset, "Quelques questions récentes sur la physiologie et la physiopathologie de la douleur" [Some recent problems concerning the physiology and physio-pathology of pain], *Presse Médicale* (May 18, 1957).

[8] Translator's note: *an-*=without, *algo*=pain, *-thymia*=suffix denoting relation to the mind, soul, or emotions.

[9] Grasset, *op. cit.*

for him that is generally admitted among "normal people." He says that he no longer feels the painful character of what we call pain, although he realizes that he should.[10]

All the more do I refuse to use the term "pain" for an animal whose brain has been removed — just as no one would have the idea of using the word "pain" for a man or animal *under anesthesia.* When anesthesia suppresses consciousness, does it not bring with it the added benefit of suppressing the consciousness of pain, that is, pain itself? The physiologist may talk of defensive behavior, or the expression of or reaction to pain, but he must do it by analogy and without trying to prove it as gospel truth. Personally, I consider that to claim a monopoly on the term "pain" for the designation of such behavior is completely arbitrary and confusing. It would be just as incorrect to use the term "suffering" to designate the participation of the psyche so essential to pain — that complicity of the cortex without which Lerich could not conceive of pain being present — and we are constrained to consider him correct.

Criticism has over and again been constructed from the mistakes of experimental analysis, and *experimentation,* like *pathology* (both precious instruments of analysis), is of real but abstract worth when it deals with pain or with any aspect of life.[11] The laboratory scientist produces signs of mechanisms and behaviors which must be carefully distinguished from pain. They may help in our understanding of pain, as long as we do not allow ourselves to be caught in the snare of abstraction and confuse the part with the whole from which it has been artificially extracted.

But we should not even speak of "a part." We are dealing with an entirely different reality, with two incomparable realities. Without gravely altering both of these realities, it is utterly impossible to look at pain with the eye of a physiologist or a surgeon, a pain amputated by narcosis or anesthesia.

The correct approach to pain can only be as a synthesis of all factors, working from the richest, the most complex, the most ambiguous, and the most mysterious of human experiences. An analysis of pain can only begin by a phenomenological treatment

[10] In reality, the lobotomized person's reactions to pain are a bit more complex. This reminds me of a delicious little story with a big lesson. A beaming patient leaves the doctor's office. "So your pain is gone?" "Not at all." "Why the big smile?" "It doesn't hurt to suffer any more." This story seems droll to us precisely because we have a sure feeling that it is impossible to validly detach raw pain from its total effects. Pain is the sum of many elements.

[11] Thus, some have defended a physiology built on reflexes, a simple but artificial unit, and so have worked up step by step to superior nervous mechanisms just as a mason builds a house.

of human pain. A simple detail can only be understood from the vantage point of the most varied study. Rather, the reality which seems most complicated to the analyst is the truth of the simplest of concrete experiences: *that pain which is the pain of all pains.*

The Unity of the Forms of Pain

If we take as our basis of study an inclusive and concrete view which progresses, not from the simple to the complex and from the bottom to the top, but from the top to the bottom and from the complex to the simple, from the richest to the poorest, then the discrimination and description of all kinds of pain — which ordinarily take up so much space — is only secondarily interesting as classification and must not detain us. The clean, sharp, quick pain of a needle; Piéron's studies in the pain of pinching and cryalgesia; the burning pain of sympathetic causalgia; the deep, lurking, indistinct pain of the internal organs; and the lightning-like pain of nerve diseases are examples of such kinds of pain.[12]

From an inclusive viewpoint, it becomes very difficult to consider *physical pain* while ignoring *psychic* and *moral pain,* difficult not to admit the close ties between *disagreeable* and *painful.* This is where I will be challenged, and it is just these fine points and this unity of the forms of pain which I wish to emphasize here.[13]

Doubtless the best way to prevent confusion is to make clear distinctions. I see nothing but advantages in calling to mind the differences pointed out between physical and moral pain, grief,

[12] Pain travels at different speeds depending on the stimulus. The sensation of touch travels at 40 meters per second, the pain from a needle at 16, from a pinch at 12, from a burn at 2 to 4 meters per second. The amyelinic fibers are responsible for slow pain. See Piéron, in *La douleur et les douleurs* [Pain and the forms of pain] (Paris: Masson), p. 38. Scherrer also has found "the distinction between sharp pain, rapidly perceived and sent along the A fibers, and dull pain, perceived after an important delay, conducted by the C fibers (Lewis, 1942) or the amyelinic fibers. In fact, the specialization of these last two groups is not so precise. Specificity of function is generally, but not necessarily, accompanied by an anatomical differentiation.* *(Ibid.,* pp. 20–22.)

[13] The desire to clearly distinguish the *differences* prevails in Jeanne Russier's short work which I have just finished reading, *La souffrance* [Suffering] (Paris: Presses Universitaires de France, collection Initiation philosophique, 1963), as over against my preoccupation with the idea of unity (cf., e.g., pp. 11, 39, 52 ff.). It is untrue, to my mind (and clinical experience as well as that of the great philosophers of suffering, such as Buddha and Schopenhauer, are on my side), that it is possible to make a clear distinction between the distressing and the painful, between psychic pain (that received) and moral pain, which *is* one's conscience ("when we deal with moral pain, we see that a man's conscience *is* his pain. . . ." p. 54). Men can get used to both of them; both of them are both received and acted.

* (end-quotes missing in French)

anguish, *ennui,* anxiety, so-called "normal" and "abnormal" pain, termed "pathological" or sick pain (which should rather be *the sickness of pain!*). But it would be a sterile effort if we left it at that and did not go beyond this diversity to recapture the *unity* of pain so clearly expressed by both language and common experience.

Dealing with the problem of *pain,* as the ordinary remark goes, is like floating on the clouds of ambiguity. We must analyze each type of pain and the particular problems of each.

But is answering the "why" of pain by an enumeration of the variety of pains not eluding the question, as Socrates ironically pointed out to Meno when he was defining virtue by enumerating virtues? Describing the forms of pain does not free us from dealing with pain itself. For pains, Socrates would say, are only different from each other to the extent that each is sharp or dull, in the feet or in the head. But "to the extent that they are all pains," they are no different from each other.

It is imperative, therefore, that we not forget the mechanisms by which pain is induced and conducted and the original characteristics of each type of pain, but we will use this information without getting bogged down in it. The richest pain certainly does not keep the most elementary pain in check, but on the other hand, it cannot be reduced to it either. Human experience demands that we approach pain in its indecomposable unity and that we question it with all the passion and demand for meaning and justification implied in the term. Scientific objectivity, cut off from human passion, can never give anything but partial explanations, abstract, and therefore false, for this experience demands that we understand it in its totality.

It is said that *suffering* is a better term than pain to express that which affects the totality of the person and requires that study deep in consciousness and time which involves my reflection, my liberty.[14] We must avoid canonizing words. Is reference not commonly made to bodily suffering; are not suffering and diseases of the organism closely associated; have some not written that the cell itself shows signs of suffering? And on the other hand, who will deny that it is completely proper to speak of moral pain, eternal pain, in the sense of sorrow and affliction?[15]

In contrast with sadness, sorrow, or unpleasantness, pain evokes

[14] L. Lavelle, *Le mal et la souffrance* (Paris: Librairie Plon), pp. 85–94. English edition is *Evil and Suffering* (New York: The Macmillan Company, 1963).

[15] The variety of meanings for pain found in Latin: affliction, chagrin, anger, resentment: *"oratio quae dolores habeat . . . detraere dolorem actionis"* (Cicero).

for the scientist a modification of the organism, at least as much a subject for the physiologist as for the psychologist. Laboratory experiments may be carried out on the pain or pains provoked by mechanical, electric, and chemical instruments; but none can be carried out on the sadness of animals. Even this is hardly true in our century of psychosomatic problems. A preoccupation with totality today has taken over the laboratories, and the study of conditioned reflexes has revealed the role of surroundings and the environment. Experiments which were thought to be isolated and pure are discovered to be impure (a change in lighting, the presence of a laboratory assistant). In short, today we avoid establishing hard and fast laws concerning artificial, experimental pain, which is, in fact, pathological pain because of the very conditions of a laboratory. It is with this in mind that I deny the existence of a pure physical pain. If it is true that man and animal are not equal in the face of pain, is this not because pain is not separable from the whole — one's race, character, or environment?

Of course physical sensibility to pain reveals its anatomical and pathological bases, its paths and its centers; we can locate its agent, the paths it follows, its speed along the nerves, through the marrow, etc. But how could we speak of the paths and centers of sadness, of sorrow, of unpleasantness, which concern the totality of the affective life and the person itself? I'm in a bad mood, I don't feel well, I'm unhappy; there is no center to locate, rather a *situation*. An outside cause can usually be incriminated, a sound or an odor. But it is usually an unknown something, a lack of comfort, a certain atmosphere, an undefinable collection of inner or outer factors. How could one confuse the sensibility and reaction to a burn with Baudelaire's *spleen*?

But if we look a little closer, we see that the limits are everywhere and nowhere. An unpleasant feeling is usually the result of a murky combination of circumstances, but occasionally its cause is to be seen in an object — that tooth which in a while will be hurting me very much. Muscular fatigue, a strident noise, a glaring light, an annoyance which was at first only disagreeable can become painful. The most exquisite pain starts as a sub-painful state which we term unpleasantness. Both pain and unpleasantness cause in us feelings of aversion, repulsion, and withdrawal.[16] Thus a biologist

[16] As we will see when dealing with the *usefulness* of pain, unpleasantness and painfulness are very close (I gladly drink the alcohol which will destroy me, but disgustedly spit out the medicine which will save me . . .). (Cf. below.)

[17] Cf. Buytendijk, *De la douleur* [On pain] (Paris: Presses Universitaires de France), p. 36.

sees in itching a weak pain, a pain in the making.[17] Because of this, no distinct line can be drawn between discomfort, uneasiness, unpleasantness, and pain.

We physicians, whose years are spent asking sick people about their suffering, asking *ourselves* what their suffering is, give the word "pain" a flexibility which includes the minutest of differentiations. In order to diagnose a stomach ailment, the physician must know the practical distinction between a heavy feeling, a burning sensation, or a cramp. We must never remove from the category of pain, of interest to us here and to both doctor and patient, that tight feeling, that uneasiness, that anxiety which is often so deadly that the deepest of burning pain would be preferable to it.

Have you been seasick? It is not a pain in the limited sense of the term. Sensations of choking, of suffocation, of tightness in the throat, of breathlessness, of asthma, of the vise-like grip of a heart attack bearing down on the chest with the terrible anguish of imminent death – all these trials drown the preciseness of pain in an abyss of pain which reaches the vital center of our existence, its roots, its nerve-center. These are no longer pain – because they have gone beyond that term and have, as it were, pushed it beyond its own perfection.

The anguish of chest pains furnishes us with another suggestive example: It shows that the boundary between physical pain and moral suffering is artificial and conventional. Of course they are each attributed to very different causes. There is no chance of confusing a friendship gone sour with a nerve disease. But the painful manifestations themselves (outside the extreme and well-localized case of a toothache, of course) show such close relations with each other. What am I saying? Their territory and objective knowledge overlap so that it is often impossible to give an exact meaning to a sharp crisis. Is there a moral reason or an organic cause?

The same difficulty with breathing, the same anxiety, the same tight feeling can come from angina pectoris, from indigestion, or from an annoyance. In the medical profession, the distinction must be made every day. Contrary to the way we may deal with the visible parts of the body (precise location of the pain, a clearly visible cause), the language of the internal organs is usually the same whether the cause of trouble is organic or psychic, physical or mental. The same thoracic pain of angina pectoris may be caused by worry or by the obstruction of a coronary artery. Some have made a distinction between "false" breast pangs and "true." It would be better to say that the "true" attack, the organic pain, may be set off by a mental problem, just as it may be caused by a muscular effort or a hepatic irritation. Anguish belongs to the world of coronary arteries and to the world of abdominal surgery — and to the world of trouble and worry.

The sudden loss of someone dear occasionally provokes such a degree of pain (or suffering) that it leads to nausea and fainting spells, but so do certain pancreatic ailments. A great sadness seems to be entirely different from a skin burn or a sting, but it grips like a grinding and pinching in the depths of one's being. Analogies between words, as coarse as they may seem, are possible because the language of the internal organs backs them up.

Thus pain and grief may both be called pain on a basis more solid than metaphor. A loss in the family does not "remind" me of a wound in the flesh; it shows itself manifestly by organic inhibition, the halt of digestive processes, nausea, vomiting, and disorders in the autonomic nervous system. There are thoughts which hurt just as much and which bring about disruptions just as palpable as a widespread burn. Body and soul are one, and the soul suffers because it is body. A moral pain is pain because it is physical and impresses itself in our flesh like a branding iron. It is impossible to imagine a moral pain outside the flesh.[18]

It is the same painful embrace which unites all the degrees of what we call discomfort, sadness, anxiety, unpleasantness, anguish, grief, smarting, suffering, cramps, burns, feelings of weight or of tightness, feelings of breathlessness or pressure. It is the same embrace which unites physical and moral man and prohibits us from eliminating one aspect or the other from our study — moral pain being fully deserving of its name since it is both mental and just as physical as the others. The same embrace prohibits us from separating the two classes of pain which we mentioned above, one biological and on the level of the individual, accessible to modern analysis, the other on a cosmic plane and accessible only to the historical or cosmo-theological vision. This differentiation of planes cannot stand up to close examination.

For the pain of a collective catastrophe can *only* reach us by individual pain, on the level of the individual. Even when multiplied and frustrated by its different forms, by the orchestration of

[18] Philosophers also recognize the unity of pain: "No pain is only physical. Every pain is moral, every pain is of the realm of man's spirit." Etienne Borne, Le problème du mal [The problem of evil] (Paris: Presses Universitaires de France, 1958), p. 11.

them all, by the collective amplitude of the disaster, the pain is always that of individuals. The carnage of war or earthquake becomes a part of the world's pain by the *intermediary* of those persons yet living who suffer in their flesh because of the dead, who become the interpreters of their woes, and who act as the tragic chorus. The world's pain is made up of the small change which the myopic physician endeavors to count in his hand. Continents are made up of grains of dust. The warnings, threats, and shouts of great historical catastrophes are always warnings, threats, and shouts from individuals. And for this reason they are accessible for biological analysis and explanation, but as the defense of a living being and as the language of aggression against the living being.

Elementary pain, like any simple element in chemistry, is the pain making up all pains. But, contrary to the elements of the chemical world, every pain lived out can contain all the pain in the world. The individualism of pain is not to be confused with its individuality. The first takes a man and his pain as the measure of the world and reduces the world to his minuteness; the other has the opposite effect — it dilates to the measure of the world and becomes the messenger and conscience of the world.

Normal Pain — Abnormal Pain: A Philosophy Under the Guise of Nomenclature

The word "pain" embraces the entire spread and diversity of those woes suffered by the living beings of man's universe. It would be impossible to take from the word a parcel of its meaning without mutilating it. Its tissue is not of a kind to be torn up into shreds. The pain of the world was cut out of one piece; it has no seams. This is why we must not allow ourselves to be entrapped in the common but far too hasty distinction between *normal* and *abnormal* pain about which entire chapters are written, but which in reality are two forms of our knowledge of pain.

"Normal" or "physiological" pain is supposed to be that which every "normal" person "normally" feels: stings, burns, cuts. "This sensation," writes Lhermite, "is known by each of us and helps us to avoid the dangers found everywhere in everyday life."[19] "Ab-

[19] Lhermite, in *La douleur et les douleurs* [Pain and the forms of pain] (Paris: Masson, 1957), p. 241. In favor of this distinction, cases of congenital insensitivity to pain are marshaled. Children burn themselves badly on a hot stove without noticing it, swallow foreign bodies into their windpipes without reacting, etc. These exceptions make the protective role of pain more prominent as well as its normalness in life. In chapter 2 we will discuss the worth of these remarks.

normal" or "pathological" pain is considered to be that which comes from an organic disorder, for example, a disorder in the very organs which sense pain, such as neuralgia.[20]

The pain of sickness, which the physician must see and combat, seems entirely different from "signal" pain (that is, normal pain) which the physiologist studies. And the argument between the two could go round and round if they were not made to understand that they are speaking of two different pains. One is peripheral, at the surface of the body; and the aggressor, the circumstances, the locality, and finally the defensive reaction may all be stated. The other is deeper, in connection with the obscurity of the internal organs and the autonomic nervous system (the sympathic system, amyelinic) ; it has connection with cenesthesia, with the psyche, with the overall functioning of an existence, including its moral aspects. This is where pain, indisposition, and anxiety may be seen in their continuity. And the break, if one had to be found for the convenience of the debate, would be located, not between physical pain and moral grief, but between the physiologist's physical pain and the pain which the doctor has in mind, between the "normal" or "signal" pain of one and the pain of sickness with which the other must engage in combat, in the midst of which it is impossible to distinguish between neuralgia and a psychological problem. Two different kinds of pain? Rather, there are two men, two viewpoints, two professions facing up to pain.

I cannot emphasize enough that there would be an immense disadvantage in fossilizing two kinds of pain. Distinguishing between "normal" and "abnormal" pain is literally conjuring away the problem of pain behind the apparently innocent smoke screen of a treatment in two divisions.

To what do these two categories, which are said "not to derive from the same principle" (Lhermite), really correspond? Should the "normal" category include toothaches and stomach cramps? Yes and no. No, because in both cases there is pathological change involved and therefore sickness. Yes, because this is certainly a case of pain normally warning us of an illness against which it enables us to protect ourselves: "It helps us to avoid the dangers found everywhere in everyday life." Yes and no: This is where the shoe pinches. Where does abnormalcy set in? Let us see.

[20] Chauchard considers that normal pain is objective, that it informs of the exterior agent which is causing it. But "internal pain, apparently spontaneous," is pathological and a sign of illness (cf. *La douleur,* in the collection *Que sais-je?* and in *Cahiers Laënnec,* no. 4, 1952) .

Toothache provides an intermediary problem by which we may slide in between the two categories "normal" and "abnormal." It is both signal-pain, because it shares in its precision, its peripheral objectivity, and sharpness, and sickness-pain, because it is disproportionate with its cause, harmful, and not definitely localized. One degree more and the toothache becomes a "rheumatic" neuralgia, often situated in the teeth, another degree more and it becomes causalgia, internal pain, or psychosomatic pain.

May we accept that sickness-pain is characterized by the disproportion between cause and effect? Everything depends on what is considered to be the cause which releases the pain. For example, the sharp pain caused by a simple touch to the skin in some diseases (peritonitis, neuritis) is termed "abnormal" (hyperesthetic). But is this pain, when the inflammation causing it is taken into consideration, not just as "normal" as a burn caused by a hot iron?

It would be better to say simply that any "normal" person suffers "normally" when he touches a hot iron, but that the heat of the iron is at the very least "abnormal." And it is just as true that any "normal" person suffering from an inflammation – no more and no less "abnormal" than a burn from an iron – will also "normally" feel pain.

Hyperesthesia is not an abnormal reaction to pain; the cause of the hyperesthesia is what is abnormal.

Should the adjectives "abnormal" or "pathological" be reserved for that pain which is "normally" (habitually) provoked by any abnormal or pathological circumstance? Is a burn any more normal than the suppuration of peritonitis or gastric hyperacidity?

Should the banality or the discretion of pain cause it to be considered "normal," with the abnormal state being considered as an excessive intensity of the normal? No one should have trouble seeing here a mobile boundary where the characteristics and variations of each person's sensitivity are of predominant importance.

We may say, then, that the distinction between normal and abnormal does not concern the different kinds of pain – in spite of the *otherwise valid* interest in emphasizing the differences between the organs of external relations and the internal organs of nutrition with regard to pain – but rather the different ways of looking at pain, the mentalities of the observers.

Any pain is *both* normal and abnormal. It is *the normal sign of an abnormal condition.* We will see in the course of this book that the paradox and scandal originate in this oscillation between the *normal* and the *abnormal* aspects of pain, an oscillation which belongs to the very essence of pain and which it would therefore be useless to endeavor to hide by an artificial division.

Is the very fact of being able to say "abnormal pain" not a revelation of the terrible confusion between the sign of the abnormal and the anomaly itself—between the sign which is supposed to warn us of evil and the evil itself? Has not the sign somehow taken the place of the evil and stolen its identity?

Has the existential (not only verbal) absurdity of these two pairs of words, "normal pain" and "abnormal pain," not struck anyone? It is ridiculous to call normal the very expression of abnormalness. And it is even more flagrantly ridiculous then to speak of abnormal pain as a denial of normal pain whose normal function was that of indicating the abnormal state. The confrontation of these two "kinds" of pain creates an incompatibility which the simple juxtaposition masked over. If we may be permitted an awkward comparison, the incompatibility is as great as that of a state whose defense mechanism has turned against it. But we had best not encroach on the subject matter of future chapters. Let it suffice that we emphasize here the importance which we see in exposing the false solution of enumerating two kinds of pain foreign, as it were, to each other, each at work on its own side so that they never meet, instead of facing up to the paradox of pain. Thanks to this simplistic division everything is easy. There are "normal" kinds of pain and there are others which are "pathological." Therefore, may we repeat it again, it is just as normal to feel the burn when one's hand passes through the flame and is injured as it is to feel burning flashes of pain when syphilis has injured the spinal cord. And it is just as "abnormal" for the flame to injure the skin as for the spirochaeta to attack the central nervous system.

The conclusion would be that the boundary is established in practice simply according to conditions of observation, the way things are seen, the degree of facility in understanding the cause of pain, the practical or experimental possibility of provoking pain or suppressing it. The causes of "abnormal" pain would be hidden, out of our reach, deeper, and more mysterious.

This is the origin of the distinction, which is common but just as incorrect, between *induced* (that is, normal) and *spontaneous* (abnormal) pain! An example of the first would be a pinprick; neuralgia (also called "essential") might be an example of the second. Doctors know well that the term "essential illness" only serves to hide our ignorance. In the same way, the term "spontaneous" illness is only an indication of the ignorance and the level of scientific knowledge for a given person or time: Those illnesses termed "essential" or "spontaneous" by our science of today will for tomorrow's scientists be induced by a very precise agent, but the illness itself is still the same. There is no more such a thing as spontaneous pain than there is a spontaneous generation! Trigeminal neuralgia *(tic douloureux)* is supposed to be "spontaneous," whereas the hyperesthesia of the surface of the stomach in peritonitis is termed "induced": an artificial nomenclature. It would be enough to "check it out yourself" to see just how "induced" and "normal" the most "essential" and "abnormal" pain really is. And if it is impossible for someone to "check it out" in person, that is no reason for him to canonize our incapabilities by making sharp distinctions.

Having beaten back a distinction between kinds of pain, one still meets a distinction between viewpoints, between levels of pain. This new statement, which may seem to be a question of semantics, in reality touches our whole problem. What is astonishing to the unlearned is not so to the scientist, and what was abnormal and spontaneous becomes normal and induced. What we thought was an objective boundary was really pure subjectivity. Better yet, this elusive boundary demonstrates the capital role played by the subject's attitude when faced with pain, especially if the pain is his.

Pain is disquieting, strange, and disarming when its cause, its meaning, and its results are all unknown. And if I notice the same uncertainty in the doctor, whom I question discreetly, then pain reaches the zenith of its "abnormalness." On the contrary, that pain whose cause (exact or not) is found easily is almost reassuring. It is "normal."[21] In this respect there is hardly any difference between physician and patient, and now we understand the chapters on "Normal Pain" and "Pathological Pain" in serious books. "Normal" pain (although it is no less pathological) is that caused by a toothache or a burned stomach after a glass of strong whiskey. "Abnormal" pain (at least for the time being) and "essential" pain, that is, that pain which seems *to incorporate in itself the entire illness,* which dominates the syndrome and which is not the sign of an illness but is itself the illness, are the terms used for certain nerve diseases the cause of which we have not as yet discovered.

What makes this criticism worthwhile is that behind a pseudoscientific nomenclature of pain, we have discovered a hidden

[21] "Is it *normal,* Doctor?" And the pain loses its interest, vanishes in thin air! Let us repeat once again that there is no objective pain, discernable to the observing eye.

philosophy. There are not two or more categories of pain which do not "derive from the same principle," [22] but two or more ways of considering pain, of reacting to it.

It is equally true that it is "normal" or "abnormal" depending on whether it meets the impassive eye of the learned physiologist, the skillful hand of the practitioner, or directly touches the ignorant and impatient patient; on whether it is common or rare, explainable or mysterious, stubborn or brief, exhausting or tolerable. It is equally true that, in obedience to the suggestive terms "normal" and "abnormal," two opposing attitudes will be formed toward pain, two philosophies – one understanding, the other rebellious, one granting, the other denying any meaning in pain.

Having beaten back what we might call a "topographical" division of pain, we meet a diversity of viewpoints, of philosophies of pain. In our opinion, the seemingly harmless nomenclature of "normal" and "abnormal" is the formulation of an *acceptance* and a *refusal* of pain.

The biologist who uses the terms "normal" and "abnormal" pain, and who considers this an expression of his neutrality, will be startled to find out that by the very abstraction of his scientific analysis he is betraying his membership in the human race. For with these terms he is speaking the common language, the philosopher's language – if it is true that the philosopher works from the language and experience of the common man – completely foreign to the scientist's abstract analyses.

Normal and abnormal are, in fact, pseudoscientific evaluations of pain. But if this division is of no objective worth, it is, nevertheless, particularly revealing as to the basis of the problem with which we are concerned. It unveils the fact that the *true problem of pain is the refusal of pain.* And from the abstract terms of the analyst, "normal" or "abnormal," we perceive as though by ricochet the true problem of pain, because this pain is a revealer of the contradiction of life and of the universe itself; because this pain is inseparable from our refusal of pain.

Pain *is* our refusal of pain. It is to be defined not biologically, but humanly, by our refusal of it. It is identical with our aversion for it. This was also the conclusion of Pradines:

> Its role (that of pain) is not to see, but to feel and to judge, that is, to feel what it judges to be evil. But for this task its very blindness is its clearsightedness. Whatever stimulant is not revealed to us by pain, no light could help us to find. It is in fact its very subjective nature which objectively gives it the

[22] Lhermite, in "*La douleur et les douleurs,* p. 241.

> nature of a stimulant. . . . What is really harmful to the organism is not a specific, exterior stimulus, nor is it any external reality, but only one subject's viewpoints as concerns a multitude of possible realities. . . .[23]

This is a profound thought which goes beyond its meaning for the biology of pain to reveal the philosophical problem of pain, that is, *the refusal of pain.* Pain has within itself a contradiction of itself, its own *negation,* with the double meaning of that term. The negation forces us to go beyond the contradiction, to progress from the level of biology to the human and spiritual plane, to reconvert the biological problem, to which science has so laboriously converted us, into the ancient problem of evil.

Duality in the Evolution of Pain

This "negation," which today we might term dialectic, is contained in the history of pain beginning with the most archaic forms, according to Pradines' penetrating analyses.

Pain was at first only a defensive irritation—just as useful as it was painless—and this is the pain that the physiologist deals with in his laboratory experiments. Defensive irritability is the first stage of a new *sense of defense,* before information from tactile (and more generally sensory) sources becomes specific and adds itself to the first stage as a sort of covering shield, more perceptive and effective in its reaction to the aggression. This "tactile shield" is therefore a secondary stage in the organism's differentiation between types of aggression. Pradines has studied its different forms which in effect substitute non-affective information, objective in the proper sense of the term (meaning that the subject places in the object the qualities which he first considered to be his own), more rapid and more precise, capable of anticipating a more distant danger and the approach of pain, for pain itself which was then deliberately relegated to a position of secondary importance.

But the result, if not the goal, of this differentiation was to consolidate and refine not only the sensitivity and consciousness of the individual as a whole, but also his sensitivity to pain itself. Paradoxically, pain regained in "painfulness" (unpleasant and even harmful acuteness) what it had lost in defensive usefulness. Its harmfulness from every point of view, and its painful quality which we know to have so negative an effect, but which were completely useless, completely foreign to the original "plan," progressively gained ground while its original role disappeared from sight.

[23] Pradines, *L'Aventure de l'esprit dans les espéces* [The adventure of the spirit in the species] (Paris: Flammarion, 1954), p. 63.

This is the form, then, that the *problem* of pain assumes in this moment of evolution which is ours. It is not a problem facing life in general; it is only for our *particular case* as superior animals, or better as civilized men.

Pain is not one of life's objective problems, but a "personal difficulty," as it were, and *only of concern to us,* or to state the same thing in other terms, *a translation of what we consider it to be.* This problem is an expression of our strange way of living and suffering pain, a pain that was not "in the nature of things," but an accident which only occurred once. But it concerns us because we have become conscious, evolved subjects, so proving Schopenhauer's pessimistic words.

For man alone — and only for some members of mankind — is pain a problem, the very problem of absurdity, the sign of senselessness, of human revolt. And basically because it really does seem to have *become absurd!*

If it were not a pleonastic statement, I would say that it is all a wonderful encounter which puts the problem into the hands of those who are capable of posing a problem! For man is the only being who sets up problems; for him justification has meaning; by him a demand for justification was born in the world; and he is the only being who questions. And it so happens that he is the one for whom problems such as pain are posed. His sensitivity and his consciousness progressed together, the one inducing what the other made into a problem. The problem of pain is the sum of all other problems since it is the general problem of justification. Would man need to justify anything if pain did not exist? It is the sum of all man's questions; it is in itself sufficient to cast the shadow of doubt over the universe.

If pain had never slapped our face and awakened us, our demands for justification, the definition of man's humanity and the keenest point of his conscience, would never have had reason for appearing. And without man's conscience, the inner drive which leads him to question and to contest, pain would doubtless never have been born either. Both exist because of the other. Pain is situated on the divide between man's biological and spiritual evolution: on the one hand, his evolution from defensive sensitivity to a sensitivity toward pain in the present sense of the word; on the other, his spiritual calling which leads him to ask questions about pain. This has been a double evolution whose components are inseparable since they are the very same thing: man's specific calling in life.

Pain represents, therefore, the typical problem, the only problem, unique — the Problem because of which all others exist, because of which everything else is a problem. Pain and problem (the problem of pain) are synonymous; pain is identical to the act by which it is contested (previously I used the word "refuse"). This is an exceptional conjunction of a particular biological situation with a special contesting power which makes man essentially a philosopher! Conjunction is an inadequate term if it is true that there are only two ways of expressing man's humanity, one emphasizing his situation, the other emphasizing the *logical* aspect of the first, its *logos,* with neither able to exist without the other. Pain and the demand for justification are two faces of the same human reality. Pain is its own problem. Pain is the refusal of pain, even when the refusal has been converted to understanding. Pain has within itself its own *negation,* which is defined by man's questionings — questionings which are already an answer in that they presuppose that man has already answered the question asked of him by the world, in that a dialogue has already been launched in which it is declared that meaning is to be found behind the apparent meaninglessness. Absurdity is no longer absurd as soon as the silence is broken. Consenting to questions about the absurdity of pain may be likened to having the obscure negative of an answer on which the question itself depends and is based. Thus, the answer precedes the questioning just as it follows — but it has changed in the meantime.

Different Degrees of Pain Mean Different Ways of Looking at Pain

There are not two or more categories of pain. There is only one pain. Viewed from one side, this understanding neither scandalizes doctor and patient nor does it incite them to any kind of war against pain. But seen from the other side, it threatens them and becomes "public enemy number one" to be overcome at all costs. This division of pain into two categories has no objective basis, but is subjective and partial, a fighting attitude, not of an individual but common to humanity: seek safety together; save your neighbor.

But, in reality, the same problem arises for all kinds of pain. The *why* when I painfully but "normally" burn myself on a hot stove and the *why* of "normal" labor pains [24] are the same as the *why*

[24] But here we have a "normal" pain which has become "abnormal," because it has been conditioned by the defective attitudes which the method called "natural childbirth," or "painless childbirth," is able to correct by creating new and better conditioned reflexes. Marxists, also, consider that most "natural" woes are "artificial."

of the fiery pains of tabes or cancer. Pain poses the problem of its own existence and of its role in every painful situation, the problem of what it has already been in each case, and of what it has meant for the sufferer.

If you take the side of *functional pain,* you cannot see why the rule is valid in the case of a skin burn or heartburn ("normal" pain), but false in the case of the intolerable pain burning through the nerves of a patient dying of cancer. And the conclusion is reached that if pain is perhaps useful in some cases, whereas it is hidden or impossible in others, the difficulty is not to be stated in terms of categories, but in terms of a transformation, of a turning upside down, of a turning inside out.

There are not two kinds of pain; there is pain. But this pain which was made (if this is the proper term) to be "normal," that is, to defend me, wandered off the track and became so monstrously hypertrophic that it became *more than* just bothersome, but dangerous, a mortal enemy for man.

"Normal" pain *does not exist* if it is to be considered as a few rare, traditional examples, always the same, in which it serves as a warning to the living organism. We do not try out the stove every day to see if it is hot, but we have learned once and for all to keep our distance.[25]

If pain is really to be defined as a defense function, how could one distinguish between useful, useless, or harmful pain without contradicting oneself? It would be better to ask these questions:

1. How can what was made to be functional pain cause us so much trouble in so many cases, to the extent that we finish by seeing in it the very image of woe, the figure of evil?

2. Why does functional pain need to be painful to complete its duty? The painful quality *sui generis* of the warning only appears necessary for the one who refuses to respect the elementary rule of Bacon's variations. And it does not take long to notice that the painfulness of the warning is assuredly a sufficient condition, but in no way indispensable. The proof of this is that the sight of pain a long way off is enough to warn us to avoid it.

However that may be, the distinction between several kinds of pain may hide, but it cannot change in any way the problem of pain. If we adopt the scientist's objective attitude, there is nothing but normal pain. If we adopt the activist, militant attitude of the

[25] A person suffering from syringomelia stays away from stoves because he has *learned*—perhaps once to his own detriment, and by education—that he will be burned without even noticing it.

patient and the doctor, there is nothing but abnormal pain (which can occasionally be providential when medical science can turn it to good use). Only the subject's attitude gives birth to this difference which some transform into "different principles."

By the same token there will be two kinds of philosophers. For some, pain is somehow "normal," that is, included in the plan of nature or creation. For others, it is "abnormal," the best argument for the senselessness of existence, worthy only of being ignored, scorned, or the object of rebellion. *But there are not two kinds of pain.*

If such is the case, before going any further in this study, we must ask ourselves not so much what pain we are talking about, but rather *who is talking about pain.* What eye is being cast upon it? Who is speaking — physiologist, physician, patient, man in revolt, believer, or rationalist? It would perhaps be even better to ask ourselves *who is qualified to talk* about pain. Who, from the list I have just enumerated, can approach the subject and understand it with the greatest measure of truth?

Before taking another step we must ask that one question, as did Buytendijk:[26] Is it the scientist, the philosopher, the biologist, or the psychologist? A scientist could only teach us the mechanisms, the *hows* of pain. But the problem of *why,* the meaning of pain, its purpose, its lack of purpose, its perverted purpose, is obviously extra-scientific. Is the physician better qualified to give a solution to this many-faceted problem, related to biology and psychology, science and philosophy? The physician, Buytendijk contends, is eminently capable of putting together a philosophical anthropology of pain which would include a general theory of corporeity and a study of the relations of men and animals with their surroundings and their own bodies.[27]

Should pain be studied biologically as a normal phenomenon or pathologically as an anomaly (which is, after all, progress over the simple division into two kinds of pain)? The physician answers this question with a politics of pain, in fact, a triple politics of pain. First, he combats it as an evil. But on other occasions, he makes use of it (although he combats it by using it) either to guide him toward a disease of which pain is the warning even though it does not itself provoke the proper defense reaction or else, when necessary, to heal, even if the remedy causes pain (although anesthesia has changed this whole picture). And, although he some-

[26] Buytendijk, *op. cit.*
[27] *Ibid.*, pp. 25, 27–28.

times uses it as one uses a turncoat, he does not gainsay that pain itself sometimes provokes false defense reactions. He must be able to detect the flaw in the sufferer and the flaw in the man who has no consciousness of suffering.

He also knows how to consider pain as part of a case history, at the end of a stage in life, and therefore as both a good and an evil – rather an evil grafted onto a good. It is both – one having become the other. He can neither conclude that pain is a good, nor that it is an evil, neither that it is a response to one of nature's "intentions," nor that it is not a response. But perhaps he can understand how it is a terrible evil, and at the same time a partial good, how Lerich was right, whereas the physiologists were wrong. The physician can understand how it is a weapon which got turned in the wrong direction – against us. And now it is doubly against us because, first of all, it is useless and occasionally harmful; second and most important, because it is unpleasant by its very *sui generis* quality of *painful* pain, which is how man knows it and experiences it. It is this painfulness which makes it *human* pain, with a brain, an intellect, a mind.

For the doctor meets *human pain.* He is qualified to speak of pain because the experience he has acquired of it is inexhaustible, unfailing, multiform, and militant. But, if he wants to penetrate its deeper meaning, he must change levels; he must become a sufferer himself, a co-sufferer; he must go beyond a politics of pain to a philosophy; he must cease being a physician *stricto sensu* in order to become a physician in the true sense of his calling; he must assume his humanity in the brotherhood-at-arms of suffering humanity.

Then the meaning of pain dominates and unites its biological sense and its ambiguity in the combat of doctor and patient. It acquires the meaning that combat gives the enemy. He is recognized as worthy of a certain respect. For the scientist, pain is "I observe, I analyze, I explain"; for the physician, "I'm against it, but I'll use it." For both of them, if they do not become converted into philosophers, painfulness is still indomitable, unidentifiable, incorrigible, and incomprehensible. But the physician, more than the laboratory biologist, is a philosopher unbeknown to himself. Whether he is fighting pain or using it, he is acting in the name of something other than action or knowledge, and the very meaning of pain for mankind is inscribed in his work. He is the embodiment of a principle of action which is the root of a philosophy of human pain. What I mean is that he shows a *preference* in his dealings with pain, a preference which has nothing scientific about it and is an anthropology in a nutshell.

When pain becomes incomprehensible for man, that step, nevertheless, brings it up to the level of the comprehensible. We can say that before it reached man, it was not comprehensible because it had no need or reason to be. *When pain becomes something else, it means something else.*

If this, therefore, is the explanation we must give of pain, it only leads to the indecision and complexity of a mixture of objective facts and ways of looking at the facts. Neither does it depend purely on the look, nor is it complete reality. Our first step must be to remove the reality from its status as an "object." We must show that this thing called pain which ambushes us, which we have to bear, and whose diversity may seem to belong to the thing itself, is due to prejudice, and, if I may call it so, to an *a priori,* to an attitude of the sufferer. We must devote ourselves to getting near to the sufferer. Diversity of pain is due to a diversity of viewpoints — sufferer and nonsufferer, doctor, scientist, or philosopher — but our task is to approach man as a collective whole, viewed as a privileged species, chosen, consecrated to pain.

Our second step is, if pain is rather in the way, to accept it, confront it, apprehend it; then actually, we end up with the old saw: *pain is what we make of it.* Pain is what we *judge* it to be (a judgment in the widest sense of the term, which includes the immediacy of the body and its functions) — evil. It is my human position which creates this fantasy, a human opinion, too human, in fact.

Yes, pain is certainly the result of a judgment, but with no intellectual pretensions whatsoever: a judgment by the body as well as the soul, a judgment which has become incarnate, imprinted in the flesh, judgment lived out, we might say — *objective* judgment. For the third step shows that our disquieting slide toward a subjective idealism of pain was only apparent. It was rather a repositioning of objectivity, from abstractness to concreteness. I am referring especially to the transfer from the disembodied objectivity of the laboratory to a new objectivity which belongs to life.

Pain was artificially reduced to the status of neutral, pure fact. But now it has been brought back from essence to existence, not so pure, not so disconcerting, and even more contradictory. It has become a fact bearing in itself its own negation and the results of that negation. Pain is itself and something else: not only in the sense that we may cast doubt on its existence, thus forcing ourselves to the trouble of clearing things up, to the trouble of an accommodation which lacks the amenities of conformism; not only, then, by our ability of contestation (our transcendental bad temper); but also in the sense that it has become an objective question, a "suspense," a *quid?*

We must emphasize this nuance. If we admit that pain has become indissolubly bonded with our judgment, we have thereby introduced the conscience into the problem, and conscience is ready to submit any and every problem to its scrutiny. But conscience is not enough here; pain would slip through only too well. For we must also admit that pain has lost its reality. It has been objectively peeled, we might say, from the sphere of reality; it has become today a problem, suspense, an objective "fly in the ointment." It is, in our sight, but also objectively (and there is no possibility of separating the two, or of measuring the part each contributes), a paradox, a dangerously bad joke. It has made an objective about-face and has become the embodiment of *refusal.*

Thus we cannot *reduce* the problem of pain to an idealistic dream (which would have the added gall of insulting the painful reality of those who suffer). Pain is an objective metaphysics, concrete, inscribed in the reality of life. Not only is it inseparably what is suffered and the doubt cast on that suffering, but this doubt belongs to the flesh itself. It cannot be removed from it; it will not let loose its grip. The result of judgment passed on the flesh, of this questioning of the flesh, is that pain identifies itself with the refusal of pain, that pain is the embodiment of refusal, of man's *no.* Any doubt cast on pain by philosophy, every verbal questioning of pain, is only a different way of pronouncing the immediate, fundamental, original *no* which is intimately a part of human reality, the salt of the human sea, that which exalts and that which kills.

Pain is the revolt of the body before moving to the mind. It is the doubt cast by the body, the judgment handed down by the body, the vital refusal of whatever mutilates and kills life. It speaks the world's woe; it is the trembling jaws of death within our own life, situated in the heart of life, devouring it alive although we hear that death and life, as some have said to console themselves, cannot be united in a face-to-face confrontation because they belong to two worlds which have nothing to do with each other. Although Epicurus would have it that when we are dead life is not there to make us cruelly desire it, with the result that we have no reason to fear an undivided situation deprived of the terror we project upon it, *pain* itself is enough to destroy the weakness of such a syllogism because it is the anticipation and almost the foretaste of death. Pain is more terrible than death itself, because we fear it twice over: once for its present sting and again for the death which it brought into life – into that life which is the very denial of pain itself, into which pain broke as an intolerable criminal, literally revolting against nature, that is, against life. Natural, and against nature, our very condition is to be against ourselves, to contain the seed of our own suicide – our own annihilation – our own death, by which we are refused the privilege of settling down. Death sends pain as its ambassador to the foreign country of life; pain is its intermediary; pain speaks the language of the land of the living although it comes from the other world. Pain is death brought within reach of the man still living, as though it were inviting him to get acquainted with the faceless Stranger. For we would, in fact, be as ignorant of death as we are of absolute absence if its messenger pain were not keeping us awake by speaking to us in our own language. That is why, as we mentioned above, man does not know if what he fears the most is suffering or dying, the negative and print of the same picture. One has color, but no sting; the other stings us so that for the moment we are over-awakened, like a leaping of flames, with the exasperation of a threatened life. But they are both daughters of the same mother; this is how we can recognize them, and the same aversion unites us against the two sisters.

A meditation on pain, then, appears as the reverse side of a meditation on death: the same questions, the same answers, or rather the same waits, the same difficulties in "hope," the same will to live beyond death, the same impossible but necessary and indispensable effort for reconciliation with Pain and with Evil.

2

Pain, an Organ of Illness

Since pain sometimes warns us of danger and sets off a defensive reflex, it would seem that it is the response to some purpose of nature. Has it a function in life, or is it a simple accident? [1] Anatomy and physiology furnish us with elements of an answer which would seem at first to confirm the common-sense opinion in favor of *pain as a biological function.*

Should we suppose that anatomical and physiological studies were to discover and to prove the existence of an organization, an organized function, even the rough outlines of an *organ* of pain, we would be obliged to admit that such an organ is somehow a part of nature's purpose – that all would *seem* to indicate that nature had prepared this organization and its function.

We would not have the idea of speaking of accident or hazard when dealing with an organ such as the eye or the ear. Their structure and their special function make it impossible to attribute them to chance. We are constrained to recognize in them a *purpose,* at least, "external."

Is there such a thing as an organ of pain? This is a fundamental question, the answer to which is more difficult in the case of pain than for the sense organs, but which nevertheless seems to elicit at least a qualified affirmative answer.

[1] Beautifully stated by Jeanne Russier: "Either pain is the consequence of an inevitable disorder, or else it is the sign of an inevitable disorder. Either I suffer in order not to die, or else I suffer because I must die." Jeanne Russier, *La souffrance* [Suffering] (Paris: Presses Universitaires de France, 1963), p. 16. But the goals and limitations of her study did not permit her to follow to the bitter end the intolerable consequences of this contradiction which it is my intention to emphasize. It also seems to me to be out of the question to treat the problem of pain and the problem of evil in different sections (p. 1), although it was inevitable in the book to which I just referred. It was no less inevitable that this principle be slighted in studying the philosophies of pain (Buddhism, etc.), and the inevitable was not avoided.

There is not *an organ* of pain in the proper sense of the term as applied to the sense organs, even in such a widespread case as the sense of touch. This statement is certainly true, but there is a certain organization, a certain systematization on the levels of anatomy and physiology of the sensation of pain. There is a certain degree of differentiation in this sensitivity, a certain specificity of receivers, of channels, and of centers — all sufficient at least to cause us to reject accident or chance as their origin.

In fact, the *nonspecific theory of pain* is no longer accepted today. According to this classic theory, held by Morat, Wundt, Charles Richet, and many others, pain is only an intensified, aggravated form of the other sensations, somehow pushed to their extreme limits. "It has no stimulus of its own," wrote Morat, "it is generally induced every time the stimulus reaches an exaggerated point which goes beyond the proper functioning limits of the organs and thereby makes its action more or less destructive of these organs." In other words, pain does not have a function of its own, but is rather injury done to other functions; it is rather, if you wish, the negative side of a positive function turned to evil, the accident of an otherwise good function placed in catastrophic conditions.

I have let myself be sidetracked by this theory to emphasize that even if it were exact, it would not change the problem with which we are dealing. For even if we were to suppose that there is nothing even faintly resembling an organization, or even the beginning of an organization, of pain; if we were to suppose that pain's only job is to express by its cries the exaggerated, abnormal, dangerous excitation of the other bodily organs, this would take nothing from its role of sentinel, the interpreter of this very situation, and the alarm sounded for the living organism. Were it to be deprived of a specific organ, reduced to the subaltern status of a *parasite* of the other sensations, pain would still occupy the position of alarm sounder when these sensations are perturbed. There is no need for an organ of pain before accepting that pain has a function, even if this function is reduced to the rudimentary cry of the threatened flesh. If, when the organ is injured, pain suddenly sprouts and grows, this is enough to attribute to it the role of a warning signal, of an alarm. What difference does it make for us to learn that this warning cry sounding the alarm of a vital danger has its own receivers, channels, and nerve centers? Even if it is deprived of any structure, of any specificity on the anatomical and physiological levels, pain still cannot be denied its reality as a sign of illness, as the language of life at bay, the elementary language of all organic suffering in the most material sense of the word: suffering as an injury done to a living cell, to living matter.

Specific Receivers, Channels, and Centers

The fact that this cry of wounded life is organized into a more or less systematic function, that it has its own receivers, its own channels, and its own centers, would not be much of an addition to what we have just said if it did not appear as a kind of backing for nature's "intention," a triumphant confirmation: "I told you so."

When we are shown that the living organism has perfected its means of reception and communication, its transmitting and listening devices, its system of gathering and conduction of information, its system of transmitting and elaborating the information into precise notions or patterns of behavior, this alarm signal is only a confirmation, with no essential information added, of the fact that pain expresses the injuries sustained by life.

With that said, the arguments in favor of the *functional specificity* of pain sensations lose much of their interest. Let us recall them, just the same, so as to remove none of the evidence in favor of the *usefulness* of pain. Its harmfulness, treated in the following chapter, will stand out all the clearer.

There is an organ of pain, but it is not definitely localized and is coarse in its differentiation. At times, it seems to be developing with the progress of life, at other times, it only seems to be an archaic evolutionary form, not following the general tendency toward a superior objectivity, precision, and rapidity of passing signals among the sense organs.

1. *Specificity in receivers.* Some experiments (such as those of Von Frey in 1896) using fine points seem to show that there are specific places on the skin for receiving pain sensations, heat sensations, and those of touch.

Goldscheider, however, thought that pain was rather a differentiation within the sense of touch. Burloud came to the conclusion, after Head's famous experiments, that the facts were in contradiction with the theory of pain as being of an archaic nature: When the trunk of a nerve renews itself after being severed, sensitivity to pain appears first, a wracking, coarse, unspecified pain, little by little dominated and replaced by touch, a more precise sense, better able to master what it is sensing, in fact capable of locating an object, of recognizing the aggressor. If pain precedes touch, it is then difficult to accept Goldscheider's theory that it is a specialized form of touch.

On the other hand, the discovery of specialized points on the skin for sensing pain would seem an easy indication of an organization of pain into an organ during the evolution of living beings.

Details on the debate may be found in the book of collective authorship entitled *La douleur et les douleurs,* for example, in the studies by Piéron and J. Scherrer. "Is pain a special entity," Scherrer begins, "or does it only represent a general mode of response by the afferent process of bodily sensations to a particularly strong stimulus? This basic problem of the specificity of pain has been discussed interminably for almost a century now." [2] "The controversy concerning the specificity of pain, as to its stimuli, its receivers (in a functional and not a morphological sense), and its channels has been established on a new foundation by the electrophysiological methods of detection used by Adrian (1932). . . ." [3]

> On the level of the integuments, Adrian and his students, Zotterman, Dodt and Hensel, and Tasaki and his colleagues were able to demonstrate a category of receivers which responded only to tactile stimulation, in this case the deformation of the integument. Other receivers responded to stimuli of a specifically harmful nature: crushing the integument or a drop of acid placed on it. *The myelinated nerve fibers, therefore, seem to select a given mode of stimulation.* Specificity is confirmed by the fact that it is possible to apply maximum stimulation to a receiving nerve fiber of touch without provoking an experience of pain or any of its outward manifestations in the animal. . . .[4]

As early as 1932, Adrian had noted the existence of receiving fibers which only reacted to pain stimuli. The conduction speed of these myelinated fibers was around 30 to 40 meters per second. Scherrer concludes:

> The extremely exact work of Maruhashi, Mizuguchi, and Tasaki (1952), carried out on isolated nerve fibers (and no longer on a fascicle of several fibers, only one of which would be active, as in the former projects), has undeniably confirmed the existence of specific fibers for the reception of pain. The diameter of these nerve fibers is from 5 to 11 microns in the cat and the frog.
>
> We can sum up by saying that the electro-physiological research carried out on animals bears witness that stimuli are undeniably received by specific fibers. A nociceptive stimulus provokes the discharge of a certain category of receiving fibers—and of one category only—the fibers of pain.[5]

[2] Scherrer, in *La douleur et les douleurs* [Pain and the forms of pain] (Paris: Masson, 1957), p. 15.

[3] *Ibid.,* p. 16.

[4] *Ibid.,* p. 17.

[5] *Ibid.,* p. 18.

There are two kinds of conduction nerve fibers for pain. Experiments have enabled us to distinguish clearly between sharp pain, rapidly perceived, conducted by the myelinated A fibers, and dull pain, perceived after an important delay, conducted by the non-myelinated C fibers (Lewis, 1942). However, the study of the electrical patterns of the latter group is infinitely more difficult and reveals a less certain degree of specificity. But, Scherrer again concludes, "The discussions around the specialization of the C fibers must not cause us to lose sight of the specificity presently well established for the myelinated fibers."[6]

2. *Specificity of channels.* Just as interesting is the specialization of the channels pain follows, the nerve fibers whose speed of conduction is slower than in those of touch. They cross in the gray matter of the spinal cord and continue along the *opposite* lateral tract, until they reach the optic lobes which might be called the diencephalon, the "between brain" of pain.

This is the place for three remarks I would like to make concerning the specificity of conducting fibers.

a) Syringomyelia (the presence of cavities in the spinal cord) demonstrates this specificity, but it also shows how rudimentary it is, how difficult it is to separate channels sensitive to pain from those sensitive to heat. In this disease they are destroyed together. It is, nevertheless, possible to distinguish within the spinothalamic tract a dorsal region which sorts out temperature sensations and a posterior region which conducts only sensations of pain.

b) The Brown-Séquard syndrome, brought about by severing either the right or the left half of the spinal cord, demonstrates the complete separation of the channels for touch sensations from those for heat and pain. When one side of the spinal cord has been severed, the sense of touch disappears on that side because the fibers of the posterior region of the spinal cord cross only at the medullary bulb. But sensations of heat and pain disappear *from the opposite side* because these fibers cross together immediately as they enter the central gray matter of the spinal cord.

c) Surgery to stop pain is a remarkable application of the specificity of the organ of pain and confirms it every day. We will deal with it in a subsequent section because it is a weapon against harmful pain, that curious other face of functional pain. We mention it here as part of our description of functional pain itself because the reality of even this "useful" pain is due to the specificity of the organs of pain. Rhizotomy severs the posterior spinal nerve

[6] *Ibid.*, p. 22.

roots between the spinal ganglion and the spinal cord. Its practice is reserved for neuralgias which follow the length of a nerve, for example, the trigeminal nerve (of the face). *Commissural myelotomy* (longitudinal incision in the spinal cord) and *cordotomy* (section of the anterolateral columns of the spinal cord) interrupt all transmissions of pain in one half of the body in certain horribly painful diseases such as cancer or tabes (a sequel of syphilis which attacks the nervous system).

These experimental and practical considerations authorize us to speak of at least a rudimentary organ of pain, for the cry of wounded living matter, which could have remained an elementary cry, seems, on the contrary, to have *begun* the undeniable organization of a system of its own. It is an unrefined organ, archaic, and, if I may propose this figure, left on the bench by the workman of evolution who devoted his time to constructions which seemed to him manifestly superior for defense. It is an archaic organ which nevertheless appears to be more developed in the higher vertebrates. Pradines, as we have seen, has clearly explained this paradox. The farther along we are in evolution, sensitivity to pain and consciousness becomes more and more refined, whereas the defense reaction which is called by the same name of pain is replaced by a new generation of instruments superior in both rapidity and precision. This helps to explain the peculiarities of Head's experiments. It is true that the regeneration of a severed nerve reproduces the sensation of pain and touch in what I will permit myself to call their genealogical order, pain then touch. But this experiment reproduces the birth of the archaic sensation of pain with the characteristics of pain that it has acquired in man. When an old pain was rejuvenated, Head witnessed the reappearance of a primitive nociceptive sensitivity (sensitivity to injurious agents) coupled with the later characteristics of pain/consciousness of which it at first had no need whatsoever. So we are endowed with a sharper sensitivity to pain than that of other living creatures at the very time when the development of other defensive factors, our senses and our intelligence, makes it useless. An accident of evolution — but its disastrous consequences have fallen on us. It is not hard to see how the discovery of an organ of pain, of useful pain, has inspired ambivalent reactions.

The Brain an Accomplice

Pain — who will disagree? — becomes keener, more complex, more refined as we "climb" the ladder of the species up to our own species. Here the observer witnesses a transformation of pain into *pain* thanks to the brain, that organ of regulation, of inhibition, and of amplification. With the appearance of consciousness man is able both to overcome his pain and also to amplify it by his apprehension, his memory, and the infinite repercussions provoked by psychological and mental factors. From that point on it is not difficult to see how inseparable are physical and moral pain.

We shall not go into the details of those functions of the brain which we have just briefly outlined. We will be content with identifying the part the brain must play in the progress of our study, for the time being concerned with grouping all the factors which contribute to an understanding of pain as a physiological function. And what is the form of this function? Receivers, channels, and centers: an architecture, an organization.

Without the brain pain is impossible, Lerich has rightly stated, and this is why we can hardly make use in our study of the experiments carried out on animals with their brains removed or under anesthesia: *Pain may not be reduced to a form of behavior.*

Pain is now only very indirectly an instrument of defense or an expression of danger. It must now be censored by the brain; it has become a *conditioned* language – in the sense of Pavlov's conditioned reflexes, it is the interpreter of an attack and the subject's total response. It has been elaborated, filtered, interpreted, socialized, and civilized.

I would like to avoid mixing the vocabulary of the neurophysiologists and the psychologists, since both are describing the same reality under two of its aspects. I would especially avoid giving the impression that I believe in the vague explanatory virtue of the brain's functions to which some reduce, at least in their method, a person's inner life. Also when I say that the brain creates the *painfulness* of pain, just as it is able to inhibit and annul the *painfulness* of pain, I simply mean that civilized man's consciousness, reflection, will, and education manifest this power of inhibition or of amplification. Nothing else, except that the integrity of the whole brain, and especially of certain parts of it, seems to be indispensable for actively exercising such a power. Saying this, I have no intention of going into the enormous problem of the connection between the brain and thought. These reservations will perhaps authorize me not to *choose* between the partisans of the corticovisceral theory (emphasis on the brain's influence over the internal organs) in the East and those in the West who belong to the psychosomatic school of thought: different schools, each with its own jargon, both explaining the same phenomena. We know that a situation influences pain, that a situation "plays the brain" as one plays a musical instrument. But we do not know how.

Thus, when the observer and the experimental scientist study the undeniable daily formation of Pavlov's conditioned reflexes, they are working with no foregone conclusion as to the solution of the problem of the connection between the psychological and the neurological aspects of action. Pavlov described mechanisms as the necessary conditions and channels without which a conditioned reflex could not be "staged." But this does not mean that the reflex is reduced to its conditioning factors, nor that the subject's interiority, made external in the reflex, may be reduced to such factors. However, we may rightly say that even this inner self is conditioned, and this in no way prejudices the problem of our liberty.[7]

We may, therefore, make use of those observations which prove the role played by the brain — of censor, of converter, of transformer, the underpinning of conscience and culture.

There is no true pain without the brain as an accomplice. As a harried traveler, I must present the long list of witnesses to this complicity without going into superfluous developments.

— One of the most popular of these signs a few years ago, under the name of *painless childbirth* showed that one of the most "natural" phenomena ("in pain shall you bring forth children") was only artificially maintained by imperfect conditioned reflexes, the apprehension acquired and transmitted from generation to generation; and that a psychological and behavioral reeducation was enough to overcome them. The pregnant woman learned and understood the *act* of childbirth, how to breathe and what positions to adopt, how to wait, and how to help the event along without tension and without allowing fear to interfere. "Painless childbirth" has been used as a war-horse by those who support the Pavlovian cortico-visceral theories, but the vocabulary of those who prefer the psychosomatic explanation has no trouble explaining it.

— In fact, the whole of pathology, not only from a psychological viewpoint, but also that of psychosomatic pathology, proves the role of the brain in the genesis, the orchestration, and the resistance of pain. Let us take as an example the paradoxical suspension of any

[7] Every step forward brings up another problem which must be set aside, but with a full realization of how much presupposition and obscurity has marked our passage. Too often we have the impression that this necessary evil is forgotten.

kind of pain in pithiatism. The sufferer from this disease is insensitive to pricking or to burning. Another example would be the phenomena of ecstasy and hypnosis in which we find the same lack of pain, the same distraction or indifference to pain. These facts provide elements for an explanation of a certain kind of asceticism, enviable and suspect, to which certain gymno-spiritual schools of the *Yoga* family would invite us. Conquer the body, and especially overcome suffering; such is the spiritual ambition of the patient techniques which make use of the brain's action on the other organs of the body.

— A more modest piece of evidence and one which puts less confidence in man is that furnished by all the illusory means of treatment which can only nourish medical scepticism: confidence, the Coué method, and the youngest of the group, the placebos — all furnish a double-edged weapon against pain since they unveil the specious quality of both pain and the weapons used to combat pain. What is a placebo? I tell you that it is no longer a placebo.[8]

The brain appears, therefore, both as the specific organ of pain, as such, and as the organ of the suspension of pain. This double action is decisive, for by it pain finds itself dispossessed, derailed from the course of its natural vocation, completely thrown out of kilter, diverted to a sidetrack. Pain becomes pain and ceases being pain. The brain (I could say consciousness and am in no way passing judgment on the relation between the two) is doubtless thwarting the original wish of "nature." Pain to such an extent transplanted, moved off-center, unrooted from its native soil, is thus emigrating to a foreign land where we no longer recognize it. It is no longer the signal closely associated with a nociceptive stimulus; it has become civilized. Debauched from the work to which its birth seems to have destined it, pain no longer corresponds to what we have learned of its anatomy and physiology. It has denied its origins and now has other pretensions, with all the risks and dangers common to "displaced persons," no matter how high they try to establish their place among the *nouveaux riches*.

The transformation of pain by, or rather at the level of, the brain enables it to attain consciousness, reflection, duration, and culture. Elementary pain reverberates through the memory, gives birth to itself by our power of anticipation, increases its dimensions

[8] Detailed experiments have shown that fake pills given instead of the prescribed medicine, with both patient and doctor unaware of the change (to insure the objectivity and impartiality of the experiment), produced a tangible, organic, and generally comparable improvement. This experiment has been carried out with sleep-inducing drugs and even with antibiotics.

in the past and in the future, and *passes under the control of time*[9] (with *infernal* eternity as its limit). It seems to be made more authentic by the notions of prognosis and duration, is strengthened and confirmed by reflection, demands an education, a civilization, a religion. Thus pain manifests its all-powerfulness by the very weapons turned against it by our technical civilization, which have become just so many sacrifices on its altar, just as the veneration it receives in the Far East takes on the virile form of *supporting* it and *overcoming* it.

We have already stated to what extent consideration of cerebral activity is insufficient to explain the leap of human consciousness by which physical pain is converted into moral and social pain. And it is just as true that the animal's psychic makeup, backed up by the brain, constitutes a veritable current reverser, if I may use the figure, and pain ceases being a pure *effect* and reveals itself to be a form of *behavior*. No longer is it only *produced by* an injury; it is produced *for* a result; in short, it is *intentional*.

[9] I will study in more detail the relationship between pain and time in chapters 2 and 3 of Part II. Some have considered that time (memory, anticipation, and imagination) transforms pain into suffering. But, in fact, time is essential to both. If a difference were sought out, it would bring the enrichment of a civilization or of a culture to bear rather on suffering than on pain. In my opinion, such names are artificial.

In any case, suppression of time does away with pain in an instantaneousness which is the perfect equivalent of *anesthesia*. It is impossible to speak of pain in animals unless this evanescent instantaneousness is verified, unless there exists in animals a certain length of duration, of anticipation, even of apprehension, of memory, of a faithfulness to oneself. It is the amplification of this faithfulness which increases and transforms pain in man, and infinitely more so in the "faithful" man ("secondary" in characteriological terms) than in a man of a "primary" character. It is sometimes stupefying to witness the rapidity with which pain is forgotten, and thus diminished, in children, weak-minded individuals, and in those qualified in psychological terms as "primary and amorphous."

I must point out in a few lines another aspect of the pain/time relationship, which has been emphasized by the psychopathologists. Compare Mme. Amado Lévy-Valensy in her thesis on knowledge and evil, *Les niveaux de l'Etre* [The levels of being] (Paris: Presses Universitaires de France, 1963). Not only does pain increase with the time on which it feeds, but *pain perturbs time*. It slows down the clock (how long the hours are when you suffer!); pain immobilizes it or paralyzes it completely. Great pain has no idea where it is in time—yesterday, today, or tomorrow. The rhythms of time are overthrown; the present is shrunk to almost nothing; the past is deformed. On its outer limits, this alienated time is cut off from time, and the abyss of the present is confused with the abyss of eternity. I no longer exist, I am dead, repeats the melancholy sufferer whose extreme pain has denied and killed his existence, his duration, his body—and space. Pain always accompanies or provokes such mistakes in time of which the first effect, and not the least important, is to devitalize time, to change creative time (Bergson's) into destructive time, which degrades both man and the world.

What does this term add to our understanding of pain, since we have already accepted that in its most elementary form pain manifests its role and function as an expression and a defense? And what difference of nature is there between this elementary purpose and that found in certain forms of pain termed "functional" which are a kind of caricature of pain swelled by a whole apparatus of cultural and social factors? In this latter type of pain the patient seeks an effect, a benefit, to be reaped from those around him. He shows by his pain that those around him are not concerned enough with his welfare, are not giving him enough time and attention. It is certainly intentional (without necessarily speaking of explicit intention) in the second degree, but it is not altered in its essence as long as its function is that of a language, an appeal in the midst of struggle, and a defense against the aggressions of life. There is no fundamental difference between the elementary cry and the psychologically sophisticated complaint. Both tend toward the same result. Although they are *effects,* they are no less *causes* and *reasons,* incitements and motives, generators of behavior and tending toward a result.

Lerich, studying certain psychosomatic and "sustained" pains, was revolted and led to hold that no one had been able to discover the thorn causing the injury: "The psyche expresses pain. It does not create it." [10] To support this affirmation, he quotes many examples taken from his long and attentive experience as a physician of pain. One patient drags himself along for years, isolated in his suffering, his face rigid, his behavior fixed in the stereotyped mold of his obsession. But those who know him agree that he used to be gay and active. Will someone not answer that his true character, at first masked, has *revealed* itself on the occasion of a conflict? This is an hypothesis that does not stand up to the proof of medicine, says Lerich. The physician's art penetrates; it relieves. The sick man changes visibly; he cheers up.

We physicians learn every day how difficult it is to get to the bottom of the origins and motives of pain. One day we have a neuropath buried in his complaints; a day later an X-ray reveals an enormous ulcer perforating his stomach. We conclude, with Lerich: Up till then our ignorance had accused him of inventing an imaginary illness. But it also happens that the same misfortunate

[10] Lerich, *La chirurgie de la douleur* [The surgery of pain], p. 108. It is difficult for me to accept that both these points could be possible: that there is no pain as long as the brain has not had its word and that the psyche does not engender pain. For, in substance, the expression of pain is identified with pain itself.

fellow, surgically healed under the best of conditions from his authentic illness, goes right on suffering and belies the surgical optimism of a Lerich.[11] Yes, it will always be difficult to assert that pain engenders a previously unknown psychology. But no one will contest this without at the same time accepting that to a certain extent the pain has simply revealed aspects and possibilities which, without it, would have remained latent. And with Lerich we accept this very complicity of the brain, so necessary for any pain to exist. In fact, it is so very necessary that in man *pain is invariably his attitude* when the brain has had its word.[12]

Pain as a Biological Function

The bodily organ of pain is a magnificent edifice if one is ready to climb all the steps, peek out all the windows. But, like some cathedrals, its building plan is a bit irregular and its final form includes some unexpected architectural features, some blunders imperfectly patched over. Nevertheless, it is an edifice. A good student could have done better, but genius is an execrable student, and nature multiplies a hundredfold the risks of genius. How many times have we conceived of a creation less imperfect than it came from the hands of the Creator!

We must take it as it is. And as it is, the organ of pain does not demonstrate beyond doubt its own usefulness.

I will not inflict on you again what I call the "hot stove argument," often the only tune that the advocates of pain know how to play. Yes, of course I am taught by pain not to get too close to a hot stove. But the strange pathological cases of indifference to pain, either congenital or acquired, are made even more impressive by the great variety of examples they furnish, as well as a sort of privileged natural experimentation on the role of pain in the life of civilized man.

[11] I am here referring to M. G. (personal observation).

[12] Concerning this point, the experience of the psychologist matches that of the neuropsychiatrist (cf. for example, dealing with those suffering from hallucinations of pain and the experience of those surgeons who are constrained to lobotomize). One who has undergone a lobotomy does not suffer from his pain, we so kindly say. But such words have a deeper meaning, both proving the complicity of the brain and casting doubt on the accepted sense of pain, since without the brain's complicity one does not suffer. Cf. chapter 1, note 18, the quotation from Et. Borne which we must complete here: "Every pain is of the realm of man's spirit and, because it hurts, it induces . . . either an effort to forget it, to escape it by diversions, or to conquer it by an objective knowledge of its causes, or else a burst of protest and revolt. . . ." Et. Borne, *Le problème du mal* [*The problem of evil*] (Paris: Presses Universitaires de France, 1958), p. 12.

A rather large number of cases have been published, cases of children and also adults insensitive to pain, a state which has its disadvantages and terrible accidents: "They are covered with scars; they have no means of defense. They burn themselves and do not even realize that it is painful."[13] They run into things, even bite themselves without it hurting. They fall and fracture a leg, then get up and walk on it. The result is seen in terrible deformations. The analysis of these facts does present some difficulty, for several anomalies are associated with the analgesia, especially a certain fragility of the bones without which the repeated fractures could hardly be explained (unless insensitivity leads to awkward movements or falls not cushioned). The negative effects are most common in childhood. If the child manages to grow up, he has learned by education that of which nature left him ignorant: how to protect himself from danger.

One report[14] deals with a thirty-five-year-old adult who had acquired insensitivity to pain after a skull injury at the age of thirteen years: While he was seated in the dentist's chair, a fine instrument fell down his throat and into his windpipe with no reaction on his part. Neither did the maneuvers involved in removing it elicit any reaction. He showed a long burn on his arm; he had gone to sleep without realizing that his arm was touching an overheated stove.

It would be useless to multiply our examples when so many may be easily found in medical reports – these cases which demonstrate so remarkably that pain does exist as a *function*. Terms are invented such as analgognosis[15] and analgothymia,[16] and these conditions are compared with the indifference to pain induced by lobotomy. And the seat of this analgesia is discussed. It is certainly not located in the periphery, but on a higher level, in the nerve relays and centers.

Our conclusion: Although the specialization of the organ of pain is rudimentary and very relative as far as the internal organs are concerned, it strikingly proves its undeniable usefulness by its pathological absence and provides excellent evidence for the thesis which gives pain its place and a definite role to play in the defense of living beings.

[13] H. Piéron, in *La douleur et les douleurs,* p. 38.

[14] A case from the files of Dr. Moreau, of the city of Nancy. Cf. P. F. Girard, et al., observations published in detail in *Lyon medical,* no. 38, (September 22, 1957).

[15] Translator's note: *an-*=without, *algo*=pain, *-gnosis*=knowledge of.

[16] See translator's note 8, chapter 1.

3

The Paradox of Pain as a Disease

An Organ of Disease, Pain Proves to Be the Disease of that Organ

There is really no sense organ of pain, but it is nevertheless somewhat organized, halfway organized, a good start on an organ meant to sense pain. And, in fact, pain has no need of an *organ* as such to assert its usefulness, as we have seen, both to the scientist and to the common sense of the man on the street, as a warning signal — a cry, an appeal, an expression, a sign, the language of wounded flesh, of an injured living being.

We have yet to ask why the injured flesh cries out. Is it a pure effect — what we might call mechanical (like one billiard ball moved by another)? Or is the cry intentional, useful, a warning to flee or to fight?

If it were purely a manifestation of catastrophe, with no finality, no intention, pain (by its very painful quality) would have appeared to the scientist to be a residue deprived of meaning; to the philosopher a revolting scandal and the very image of evil. But such is not the case, and *the channel leading from the problem of pain to the mystery of evil deserves not to be short-circuited.* Throughout the first chapter, pain showed its titles and diplomas, its manifest goodwill and good faith, and we took good care not to scorn such evidence. More than a casual servant, it shows us its plans, its systematic and organizing spirit.

As the spontaneous expression of a harmful situation, pain has demonstrated its *intentional* character. Moreover, as we have already remarked, submitting that an expression is intentional is really only a stronger statement of the word "expression" itself. Blondel has written very correctly that

> the inner unity of an expressive phenomenon is its intention, but an intention already on its way to realization. . . . There is a relationship between the natural expression of an act and the more or less intentional goal of that act. The language of the emotions is the spontaneous first step toward satisfying needs or warding off dangers. . . . There is nothing, therefore, which is not

part of the voluntary plans of our life, nothing which does not serve them, not even the spontaneous manifestations of our most intimate processes or the expressive unity of an act.[1]

There is no expression which is not intentional. Even if pain were deprived of any official function, it would conserve its function as an expression.

The fact that pain is the expression of an evil which is attacking me does not do away with two questions: The first concerns the ill itself; the second concerns the ill that this expression, because it is painful, brings with it as though it were an extra treat. A third question may be added to these two if the expression itself is seen to be an intention as well as the defense. If, according to Blondel, the expression of the illness and the reaction as flight or struggle are the same thing, nevertheless the expression often wears out the reaction. Instead of stimulating it, occasionally it seems to stop it cold. There is a big step from pain as an expression to pain as a defensive reflex, at least as far as its effectiveness is concerned. And this step must not be ignored when considering the usefulness of pain.

In our examination in this chapter of the defects and mistakes of pain as a function, our main task will be to measure the distance between these two modes of pain's intentionality: is it only an expression? Or is it only an effective defense?

An Erratic Ally More Dangerous than an Enemy

We have already seen our subject of pain to be an effective defense agent. Happy is the wounding, burning touch, happy the toothache — for the one who immediately profits by the experience! Happy also is the animal who carries its own quills or other protective armor to ward off the aggressor or to discourage it from coming back for more. Defense as a warning to the sufferer is backed up by defense as pain inflicted on others.

But, besides these undeniable assets, how many times has our ally been proved at fault! The file of accusations would soon overflow with condemnatory banalities if we did not take care to interject a critical note.

It is not rare to see a serious danger threaten someone without his being warned by pain: a cancer develops; tuberculosis or syphilis progresses. A stomach ulcer, usually painful, sometimes reveals itself by dangerous internal hemorrhaging without previous warning: not the least cramp, neither to warn us of the illness, nor to

[1] M. Blondel, *L'Action* (Paris: Presses Universitaires de France, 1893), p. 209.

indicate that the hemorrhaging is really caused by an ulcer and not from an etiology requiring an entirely different treatment.[2] If pain always pointed out the coming danger, there would be no such thing as "too late!" There would be no insidious beginnings with falsely innocent appearances which disquiet no one. And a confused signal is not much better: a simple heavy feeling in the stomach may hide an indigestion, a cancer, or a heart attack.

Allow me to interrupt momentarily this benign explosion of resentment. Of what are we really accusing pain? In the first case, of not staying at its post; in the last, of lacking precision. These are two entirely different accusations. It is a remarkable reproach, flattering to a servant, that of being missed at an opportune moment; is this not a double proof of pain's indispensable nature? Our resentment must not go so far as to confuse the case against pain with that against non-pain! This would only be an homage rendered by inadvertence.

More precisely formulated, the lack of pain's signal is in reality confused with its lack of precision: The first lack disappears in the second. We are not so much against the absence of pain as against pain which arrives at the wrong time, without rhyme or reason. If there were no pain, well, we would just have to get along without it. But our nature is so formed that we are accustomed to counting on it; and no matter how undesirable pain may appear to us, it is even more so if it does not appear when it should.

Let it suffice us, then, to learn not to ask of pain more than it can give us. When it warns, so much the better (or so much the worse), but we must learn to *anticipate* it and as often as possible to get along without it. Is it not the role of what we call *preventive* medicine to track down the ills against which pain does not warn or has not yet sounded a warning?

We cannot trust pain; we must not make it the guardian of our health or of our lives. The reproach made to an ally of being missed during his absence may be friendly, but the same reproach made to a sentinel, whose job was to stay at his post, is entirely different. Learning not to count on someone is not regretting just an occa-

[2] The problem of severe hemorrhaging in the digestive tract is one of the most delicate faced by a surgeon under the pressure of an emergency. One kind requires surgery; the other absolutely contraindicates it. The problem is to distinguish between them, and if the condition is due to an ulcer but the pain so characteristic of that disease is missing, pain's absence is cruel. In that case, the ulcer goes right on bleeding without identifying itself. Is it an ulcer? Or is it another hemorrhagic disease somewhere else in the digestive tube? Not only the diagnosis, but also the patient's life hangs on the correct answer.

sional absence; it is considering *both* his presence *and* his absence to be faulty. A careless ally brings on more dangers than the enemy, and pain is not so much at fault by its absence as by its inconstancy.

A dog with a broken leg avoids putting any weight on it, and pain thus becomes the ally of healing. But a horse puts its weight on a wounded leg, and this is what keeps it from healing. Some have cited the case of an insect which devours its own entrails without the slightest knowledge that they are its own — all that is necessary is to put them between his mandibles. Other lower animals go their way, with no qualms at leaving half their body behind. These examples taken from the animal kingdom prevent us from claiming that there has been some unknown degeneration of a natural sense of pain in man (Burloud).

Excessive Pain Supplants Illness Itself

In contrast with pain as a warning, in which case everything seems to indicate its necessity, there is the opposite extreme: an intense, excessive pain, out of all proportion with the ridiculous or nonexistent danger we are in. No one will deny that a raging toothache, whatever its usefulness may be, is only sounding the alarm for one sick tooth, which is not a threat to our lives. The smallest cavities are sometimes the most painful. Pain here has already taken on more importance than the lesion, so much so that it may become *the only reason for treating the lesion.* Pain has replaced the illness, has taken its place, has become the illness itself.

A few more examples: An attack of biliary colic warns me in its own way that I have stones in my hepatic duct. Pain has, of course, sounded a warning against the lesion, but I must add immediately that *the lesion is only a lesion because of the pain!*

Enormous kidney stones silently threaten a life; the smallest ones, by their progress and the very fact that they are so small, provoke terrible colics. It is even thought that the intensity of the pain impedes the progress of the stone, slows down its expulsion from the urinary tubes, and by the paralysis itself and the spasms of the canals prolongs the torture and retards healing. It is a vicious circle, which we must treat in more detail later, but for which pain seems to be directly responsible.

A pain incomparable to the danger incurred ends up becoming its own danger. An ally turns against the one it was supposed to serve.

The neuralgias — facial, sciatic, anal — are so severe as to make us think of suicide. But they have no important, vital function (which does not mean that they have no function whatsoever). Thus we are led from excessive pain to *dangerous* pain. Now it is far from providing useful but awkward, clumsy indications of a sickness to be treated, of a danger to be warded off. Now it forges ahead of such bumbling varieties and usurps the name of illness, takes the place of the ill that it was supposed to help us fight, and becomes THE ILLNESS to be fought off, the only one, the most terrible one, the great enemy of patient and doctor. Instead of helping us in our battle against illness, it makes the illness worse, impedes our means of defense, paralyzes us, throws its hand in with the injury which it is prolonging and making more rebellious, more difficult to reduce.

To warn of sickness there is pain, but what shall we do when the cry of pain is the sickness itself?

There is no lack of examples of cases where pain prolongs the illness, becomes an obstacle to the physician trying to interrupt its course. Several lines ago I used the example of the minute stone in the ureter responsible for the spasms of pain which block it and immobilize its progression toward the exterior, which prevent it from expelling itself and which thus prolong the pain itself and its results. The anal fissure will not heal as long as it causes pain. So, infiltrating the fissure with an anesthetic liquid is often enough to stop its progress. At the best, no attention is then paid to its healing over, and the physician is sometimes surprised to find the fissure still there several weeks later but causing no pain to the patient who is completely unaware of it. It was not the slit itself which he feared; it was the pain which was important. He thought that by removing the pain, the fissure would go away also. It almost seems that nature (to give a name to the impersonal "it") went so far in its cynicism as to be scornful of any longer hiding the pain under the disguise of a lesion and, once the trick was discovered, did not even take the pains to hide the evidence.

Strangulated hemorrhoidal thrombosis and strangulated hernias grow and tighten the bonds (like an animal taken in a net) of their own incarceration. The more the edema swells and the painful collar tightens down, the more resistant they become to any manual treatment. A sprain, once it has been infiltrated with novocain, is ready to go again — which proves that it was only the pain and not the injury which was preventing its action a moment before. Nevertheless, it would have swelled up and immobilized its victim for several days.

Here we must be careful! I fear that by means of an association, or a figure of speech, pain will be accused of the evils which should be assigned to the agitation of nerves and hormones which accompanies pain. The difference between the two may seem small, but it is important and if not distinguished would deprive us of an essential piece of evidence.

In spite of the parallels which exist between them, it is important not to confuse pain and manifestations of the autonomic nervous system. I say "parallels" with a partial comparison in mind with what goes on between the mind and the brain. For the difficulty is the same. We are both authorized and forbidden to identify the two – the psychic etiology and the organic etiology, experienced pain and the disorder of nerves and hormones. Lerich, by treating the sympathetic nervous system with his infiltrates, was actually working on both sides, and the benefit realized on the level of the autonomic system was attributed to the disappearance of the most striking symptom, pain. The confusion is due to the fact that it is the agitated nerves and hormones (there is no need to distinguish between the two at this point) which are exacerbating that pain which is only a symptom. Thus, the slips today generally recognized in the process of alarm and defense proposed by Selye, mistakes as far as the organism is concerned, are not necessarily mistakes as far as pain is concerned. For if pain is part of our defensive "arsenal," the entire arsenal is not summed up in that one weapon. It is no less tempting to try to blame everything on those people who, like the cock in a fable, crow at the top of their voices without worrying about who hears them. In rheumatism, the disorder of the defense system is guilty, not the pain which accompanies it; analgesics are less effective as sedatives than by their influence on hormonal reactions. Aspirin is today called the "poor man's cortisone." [3]

It is said that pain obstructs the defense system of a living being. And the phrase catches on; it evokes an animal literally frozen in its tracks, unable to attack or to flee. But it is only an image. "Traumatic shock" is a clear example of an "obstruction" of an organism all out of proportion with the injury involved. The victim may die as a result. However, if he can be helped over the hump of this obstruction (by the techniques of extreme cold, among others), he is saved. Are we dealing with pain here? On the contrary, the shock here is anesthetic in its effect, and it is the

[3] Aspirin, the classic analgesic; cortisone, a medicine belonging to the family of hormones (produced naturally by the glands of internal secretion).

absence of pain which shows that the victim is no longer fighting. We can see, then, that pain must not receive too much emphasis, neither too little: an epiphenomenon in a tragedy which is much more important than this simple symptom, when present is nothing, when absent even less, since once again it is absent from its sentry-box.

Another favorite image is that of the prey "fascinated" by its tormenter. But I have put too much emphasis on the snares of arguments based on analogies between animals and what we experience not to remark concerning this figure that a "catastrophic" behavior would seem to be inspired by fear, that it resembles what we men experience in paralyzing terror, but that such a resemblance cannot stand in place of proof. An analogy only proves the analogy.

I would not be so hard on the identification of pain with terror. The relationship is close between the anguish which paralyzes in the face of danger or even throws the maddened man or animal into the face of danger, and pain in the narrowest sense. Terror is pain stretched to the limits and roots of life, and in the introduction to this book, I prepared the ground for an acceptance of the difficulties involved in this kind of terminology. But it would nevertheless be proper to ask of me some examples of physical pain alone as a paralyzing agent, inhibiting the organism, preventing it from warding off the danger. Such examples will not be easy to locate, for hesitation will always be possible. Is the obstacle pain itself or is pain only organizing a spasm, a sympathetic inhibition responsible for the immobility called "terror" (or "pain")?

Is it anger that makes a cat's fur stand on end? Or rather, is it the opposite? According to physiologists, an injection of adrenaline will make the fur stand on end and produce anger. Parallels and epiphenomena meet us at every step and could put us on a sort of treadmill. Let us take another look at my previous example of an anal fissure. The infiltration of an anesthetic causes the pain to disappear and *at the same time* provokes sympathetic and local vasomotor modifications. Just because the doctor directed the anesthetic against pain does not mean that the healing was accelerated only by the disappearance of the pain *(post hoc . . .)*.

So truly conclusive examples of disrupting pain can only exist on the level of human psychology, when by its brutality pain prevents us from moving, from defending ourselves. Will we never know, then, whether it is the pain or harmful modifications of the organism which stop us in our tracks? Let us not become ensnared in the confusion which is so frequent, as we have already pointed out, between behavior due to pain and the pain itself. We could make ours these words of Pradines concerning the confusion "between the useful effects of pain [which, by the way, he challenges] and those of the motor aversion which accompanies it. This aversion is undeniably of a rather adaptive nature, and its ordinary effect is to avert a harmful agent. . . . But its adaptive nature may not be seen in the consciousness of pain which accompanies it."[4] So the harmful nature of certain forms of behavior, of certain reactions, may not be seen in the pain which accompanies them. What was taken as a flaw in the chapter on useful pain may be used in its defense in the analysis of the proofs of its harmfulness.

The conclusion of this examination is that it is impossible to furnish a conclusive example of aggravating pain without running the risk of imprudently confusing it with the nervous and hormonal disorder which goes hand in hand with it. Pain may paralyze our psychological reactions, may stop us from fleeing. But let us say, rather, that it is contemporaneous with the body's inhibiting reactions. It does not provoke the spasm or the immobility; it is only a witness.

Considering our progress so far, it would be difficult not to feel that our accusations have mostly been losing ground, if we may think of pain as on trial, and that this general retreat of our accusing arguments has almost brought us back to where we started.

No, we cannot charge pain with all the mistakes of our defense system. Neither, as we must also accept, can we decorate pain for the benefits that the defense system affords. It has been shown that the speed of conduction is lower in the pain fibers and that, whatever other meaning this may have, the information takes longer to reach the consciousness and warn it than it takes the body to react to the aggression. Thus pain is much less of a warning signal than an accompanist. It *follows* the defense reaction (termed "the behavior of pain"), *instead of provoking it.* The behavioral reaction can take place without pain since it leaves before the pain arrives. Pain is more of an expression than a mobilization.

The conclusion of our analysis is that pain, in the mistakes of the defense system as in its successes, does not help bodily defense any more than we can say with certitude that it inhibits it,[5] *but it*

[4] Pradines, *L'Aventure de l'esprit dans les espèces* [The adventure of the spirit of the species] (Paris: Flammarion, 1954), p. 129.

[5] "Many experiments have shown that if, in its moderate forms, pain may produce some sthenic effects, its development always entails asthenic and even mortal effects. The absurdities of pain have provided material for all the recent literature on the question." *Ibid.*

does end up as its own greatest disadvantage. If we were to suppose that everything would go on without it, both on the positive and negative sides, its disadvantages far outweigh whatever advantages it may have. If we were to suppose, on the contrary, that we had been able to prove its effective participation in both happy and not-so-happy defense reactions — which is not the case — the collection of pain's misdeeds would have been more than adequate to cancel out its benefits.

The Physician's Hand-to-Hand Combat with Pain

We will drop, therefore, our references to pain as an aggravating factor in danger and will be content with a position less advanced but solider. Even if only pain's "stressing" effect is retained (Selye defines "stress" as any alarm of an organism), and if we reduce, as I have already done, its disadvantages to the major disadvantage of its own existence, it is no less in its own right a heavy handicap, an *illness,* perhaps the most frequent and the most terrible illness that we have to combat in man.

Although we probably must no longer hold that sickness is healed by applying an anesthesia to the pain, it may be very solidly proven that the doctor's task is to care for both the disease in question and the pain which often takes on so much importance that it may, as the outer limit, itself constitute the illness. Neuralgias would be one example of this category, for to treat them, all the attention is given to cutting off the channels of pain by drugs, surface applications, or even nerve sections.

There is what is called pathological pain, subject matter for a chapter, as we have already mentioned, in the books on pain, usually entitled "abnormal pain," or "pain as an illness," considered as the opposite of what is not without humor called "normal" pain. But whatever its baptized name, it is somewhat strange to witness, after our long discussion of pain as an organ of illness, that there is an illness of this organ.

There are illnesses which are centered, concentrated, and summed up in their pain, which are pain and nothing else. In such cases pain does not play the part of an expression or a warning of danger, but is itself the danger.[6]

[6] The well-known specialist in clinical medicine, Paul Savy of Lyons, has written in the introduction to his *Traité de Thérapeutique clinique* [Treatise on clinical therapeutics]: "Pain itself requires to be treated. Secondary phenomena, multiple reactions both physical and mental, the vicious circle of suffering prolonging suffering can and must disappear under treatment with analgesics. . . ."

If someone wants to gather information on man's struggles with pain, he should speak to a physician: He knows what he is talking about when it comes to pain.

Pain for the physician, and the paradox of medicine dealing with pain. Such could be the title of this chapter.

Pain is considered to be the doctor's helper: "The young Bernard J. . . . was just saved at a friend's place from acute appendicitis. Just in time. Without the pain, would they have saved his life? The classic rule prevents me from giving morphine to stop an abdominal pain which may hide a future appendicitis attack. Is this not the proof that pain is useful and must be respected?" [7]

This is true in some cases. But in most, our sentinel transmits blurred indications which are unprecise, false, rather made to lead astray than to guide.

Much could be said of the whimsical directions given by pain to the searching doctor. Burning pains in the stomach are obvious abdominal signs. But the illness could be pneumonia in a child or camouflaged nephritic colic. An indigestion seems to lead me to the digestive tract; in actual fact it is an attack of angina pectoris. "The central fibers of the long reflexes do not correspond in number to the peripheral fibers. This is why pain of the internal organs may not always be located precisely." [8] It is therefore impossible to expect the same precision in the channels of internal pain as that reached by cutaneous pain. We are only too well acquainted with pain as a ventriloquist, a scout leaving false tracks. Its sensitive spots are often only of interest to the young novice physician who lets himself be taken in.

The physician's wary attitude toward pain should make us stop and think. He uses its information, but stays on his guard. What good would his technical formation be — his flair, the tricks of his trade — if his job were not to discover the snares laid for him by pain? And all this goes on just when the patient and the onlookers naively imagine that it is enough to be guided by it. They find it hard to understand why doctors resist the temptation to answer the "message" of pain in its own language. The patients believe

[7] This remark was made to me. We must note that the lack of precision in the pain had once again led the doctor astray and retarded surgery for four days, without in any way hindering the acute attack. And the fact, I added, that *we use* pain does not make pain *useful* for anything. We have learned to use an attack in the lower right abdomen as a means of discovering appendicitis, but what Bernardin de Saint-Pierre would intimate that pain was intended for such an usage? (Cf. translator's note 2, p. 80.)

[8] Gruner, in *La douleur et les douleurs,* p. 11.

its very word and take it at face value: "I have a stomachache (personal diagnostic); I am going to consult a stomach specialist; I want a stomach X-ray and a treatment for my stomach. . . ." The poor fellow, he was suffering from something entirely different, gallstones, for example, or professional worries.[9]

The physician finds in pain an unsure ally and often a false witness. He uses it when he can and as he can, in those cases, of course, for which it gives him some sign, a sign which he must put through the crucible of his criticism. Sometimes he has to keep the pain quiet — a raucous static that deforms and drowns out the objective symptoms as static disrupts a radio broadcast. Finally, just as pain disturbs an objective examination, it impedes surgery: *what would we do without anesthesia?*[10] It does not happen less frequently that the therapeutist is constrained to cause pain in order to treat and heal, a fact that should set us to thinking. For someone who is curious about the ambiguity of pain, is it not strange and just a bit paradoxical, that the same man who is responsible for soothing pain is yet liable to have to cause pain for my own good? Think of all the disagreeable items, large or small, exploring instruments and hypodermic needles (even the shot given *to put pain to sleep!*), which give the doctor and the dentist such a sad reputation! The children are not the only ones to wriggle when they see a doctor's white coat. They know what is afoot. Is

[9] The ambiguity of the information furnished by pain was a problem for a *Colloque sur les problèmes de la communication* [Colloquium on the problems of communication] (December, 1960), two volumes published by La Documentation Scientifique. I will quote a few lines from that report: "An illness, a symptom, pain: all coded messages received by the doctor, which he must decipher. Such is his profession. First, he must begin communication with the body, an enigmatic body which expresses itself through blurred signals, confused signs, better meant to lead astray. To tell me that a mortal heart attack is about to sweep me away, the body stammers out a vague indigestion. A major and necessary task would be to elucidate the snares inherent in the language of pain. . . . Discomfort often deviates from its organic source. Often it is the expression in an organ of some psychological conflict—the visible symptom of an invisible problem. Communication then requires a *double translation* in order to work its way back up the winding path which leads first from the apparent symptom to the real disorder, then to the problem of life expressed in that disorder. A medium of double refraction. A double criticism of the testimony borne: the body's illness is critically examined by the symptom; but even more important, the problem of life must undergo the criticism of the body's illness" (J. Sarano, *Communication et communauté humaine de santé* [Communication and the human community of health, pp. 470 ff.).

[10] I am not saying that there was no surgery before anesthesia. People did not use to be so timid in the face of pain. But the fact that the suppression of pain permitted the extraordinary progress of treatment by surgical operation is less in favor of pain's usefulness than of its harmfulness.

it not a bit laughable that the man devoted to stopping pain is the very one we are apprehensive of visiting, because he will hurt us to heal our hurt?[11]

However that may be, *pain is so ineffective as the sign of an ill that it has now changed its signal.* It has often been repeated that pleasantness and unpleasantness are poor judges of usefulness and harmfulness. Pain is beneficent; it sometimes saves from injury or death, whereas its opposite, pleasure, is the gate to perdition (sobriety! no alcohol, no pastries; exercise, so tiring that we huff and puff and perspire to the point of "feeling ill"!).

Pain is the healthy warning signal of illness? Come now! It is indifferently a sign of good and a sign of evil, without counting all the cases — and here I return to my subject after this long digression on the rather contradictory relationship which exists between pain and the physician — *in which it appears itself as the worst evil.* But I do not want to leave my digression without remarking (as an anticipation of what we have yet to study) that *pain as a useful trial is a most humorous reverse side of pain as the alarm signal against mortal danger.*

The Patient's Hand-to-Hand Combat with Pain

After pain as an expression of evil and in its own way a first step of defense, and after pain as a healthy operation which is the very opposite of the mortal danger it is pointing out, follows that pain which is a mortal danger in itself. We have studied the doctor's relationship with pain; now let us study *the relationship between the patient and his pain.*

In an illness, the most tyrannical feeling, and that from which the patient wants most of all to be delivered, is pain. A night attack of colic: nephritic? hepatic? First a shot, and unless there is a risk of appendicitis, the physician called in an emergency starts by soothing the pain of the attack. He will come back tomorrow for the diagnosis, maybe never. Once the pain is gone, it is easy to forget that an etiology was behind the pain, capable of causing its return. The repetition of painful attacks will invite more thorough examination. In short, the sickness was summed up in the pain as far as the careless patient and the superficial physician are concerned. They do not go much further than that, but their identification of the two is nevertheless evocative. For

[11] Psychiatry has had much to say about the original ambivalence of the doctor/patient relationship. Compare the work by J. P. Valabrega, *La Relation thérapeutique* [The therapeutic relationship] (Paris: Flammarion, 1962).

if pain is a weapon for the organism, how is it possible that patient and physician must arm themselves to combat it?

The day-after-day effectiveness of "symptomatic" treatment of the most diverse ills, however unsatisfying it may be to the scientist concerned about etiologies, is nonetheless sufficient to raise the question, *"Who* is this ally we call Pain?" We spend our lives worrying, not so much about how to avoid it (which would only be a proof of its usefulness) as how to combat it face to face!

But, someone will say, do we not have to protect ourselves against defects in our most indispensable organs, against their own illnesses which turn them against themselves, and against the men for whom they are life itself? Should we be surprised, then, to see the same thing happening in this defense organ?

This remark would be valid (we will study it in detail in the next chapter) if pain were an organ like the others. But it is not. Its very existence is *by* and *for* illness in the other organs. Pain is supposed to give voice to their ills, and it is difficult to conceive of pain itself being ill. How to picture *the pain* of *pain*? [12]

If pain is what announces to the earth and its living beings what is disrupting and threatening life, what will warn of its own disruption, of the fact that it is itself threatening us?

– "How naive!" someone else will retort. This is no harder to imagine than that the professional himself, the physician, may some day be sick himself, just like everybody else!

– The very idea of a sick doctor does makes us smile, as though there were in his illness something vicious, something ridiculous, which inspires in the depths of our soul the fear of an almost anti-natural anomaly rather than the satisfaction of a patient being avenged of his tormenting doctor. An illogical reaction, probably, but meaningful. But let us not anticipate the next chapter.

To get back to the identification of pain and illness, we must admit that such an identification is too simple. And we must recognize that pain and illness are no longer confused by those who understand (and no medical course is necessary) that there are illnesses which are much more important than the pain which may or may not embellish them.

[12] It could not be stated better than in these words: "An alarm system . . . a bell, for example, which is supposed to ring automatically to warn of a fire or a robbery, does not itself produce a small fire, or a robbery. But the sadness with which we react to certain events, fear or anguish, not only signals certain woes, but is itself evil. We are dealing here with a system which, in order to warn of an evil, spreads another evil" (L. B. Geiger, *L'expérience du mal* [The experience of evil], p. 42).

Without confusing lesion and illness, and while emphasizing that illness does not do away with the category of lesions,[13] "pain" must be given a very wide range of meaning, as I tried to do in *La Guérison:* "the importance of defining a morbid state by present or future suffering." [14] This is doubtlessly true if, in one way or another, any *functional diminution* (in the sense that a man is *diminished)* is felt as pain. I wrote then that this was a "totally functional" definition of pain, rather than what could properly be termed a *subjective* definition, although it is impossible to "separate these two expressions of a single criterion with regard to the subject." [15] The term "pain" sums them up since it is valid for every mutilation of our capacity to live, of our creative activity, of our power to win out in difficulties and to adapt to situations. "Subjective" and "functional" are closely united when the functional diminution meets a poor reception; but, as we know, it is often accepted with indifference or even secret pleasure, so the above comparison must not be too closely pressed. *Functional diminution,* which we believe to be a definition of sickness, is what we might call a mixture of inner and outer factors, with a subjective face and an objective, the subjective face corresponding to pain in the widest sense, a diminution felt to be such.

Sickness may not be identified with pain, but pain represents

[13] Cf. J. Sarano, *La Guérison* [Healing] (Paris: Presses Universitaires de France, 1955), p. 16. One of the snares of medicine is the innocent lesion which becomes the object of every attention: "Heart murmur, an anomaly which shows up in an X-ray, a malformation of a bone, gallstones, etc., which will never bother the patient: are these illnesses?" Other examples are given which show the role of pain as an intermediary to transform a lesion into an illness (see note 14, below).

[14] *Ibid.,* p. 17: "We may call unusual cardiac noise or high blood pressure pathological, but because of the lack of breath or the discomfort which the subject experiences. Without being ill, such a person is on the waiting list for, and is liable to, illness and must be treated or observed. . . . As for the sick person who is unaware of his illness, he is also unaware that he is liable to suffering and that some day soon he will be suffering. It is only because of this future that he may correctly be called sick. Admitting rather that by certain signs *I foresee that he will be sick* is avoiding a rash confusion of lesion with illness and is justifying the phrase 'preventive medicine' (or the task of recognizing a disease by its first signs). Macroscopic, histological, radiological, or humoral alterations have no real meaning except by the very relative degree of prediction which they afford (like the weather bulletin in meteorology). Of course, the doctor has the right and the practical duty of seeing an illness behind the objective appearance of someone who is not in pain, and of acting early. But the very dangers of such predictions show that their foundations are very approximative, and we sometimes operate on an anomaly which is responsible for nothing."

[15] *Ibid.,* p. 24.

the heavy sword which weighs down one side of the balance and takes priority in deciding when illness is present and what treatment to apply. Pain is an expression of the *functional difficulty* which is properly termed illness. But most important, even if illness is not always pain, pain *is* illness.

"Pain is sickness," Lerich repeats, and the joint experiences of patient and physician practically always prove him to be right. Not only is pain sickness, but it is the most frequent, the most fearful of illnesses, and the physician's task is henceforth to wage particular war against it. The doctor must concentrate his efforts against it; it becomes his *bête noire* — his number one enemy.

What possible good can such terrible pain do for the dying victim of cancer, a pain which only sick humor could still call a defense function? What good can migraine headaches do, sciatic or trigeminal neuralgia? The therapeutics of pain, becoming more important every day, furnishes the irrefutable proof of *pain as an illness,* whereas we thought it was a *sign* of illness, helping us to defend ourselves from our illness.

Is it not strange, then — and this conclusion will lead us to the next chapter and a study of all the facts we have gathered together concerning pain — is it not strange to see this function of a living being, seemingly intended to warn us of an enemy's approach, become itself the enemy? Pain is not only an awkward, excessive, invading (save me from my friends!), dangerous helper, but the ally who turns his back, the traitor, the one who leads me astray, who wounds me, and who finally kills me. The *organization* meant to defend the living being (which I was rather pleased to describe in chapter 2 as to its architecture, blueprint, anatomy, and physiology) has turned against us. A weapon to combat illness, now it must be combated itself. Instead of an expression of illness we now find ourselves faced with the expression as an illness. The organ of sickness has become the sickness of that organ. The signal of illness has itself become illness, a danger in itself. Not the signal of danger, but the signal itself a danger — this reversal forces us to think, obliges us to reconsider the problem. Like a scorpion its stinger is turned in toward itself. What monstrous lapse of nature and of life is this confronting us? Have we not the right to look on this organ with the same aversion we feel for monstrosities of nature, *for acts against nature*? Would it not be correct to call pain the "first suicide," the "original suicide of life," and the truest indication of the existence of a radical Evil in the heart of creation?

4

The Reversal of Pain

We are dealing here with two faces of pain, not with two distinct kinds of pain. It is true, then, that pain does sound the alarm when danger threatens life, and it is true that it in turn becomes a dangerous weight. It is true that *pain purports to exercise a function,* but it is also true that it provides the negative spectacle of an absence of intentionality — an accident, a desertion, a rout, *the negation of any functional worth.* Thus we are asserting both aspects of pain, or two kinds of pain, when we are satisfied with emphasizing first one point and then the other, or with accepting both at the same time. Pain for some is like the tongues served by Aesop, at the same time good and evil.

Such an attitude fails to understand that a juxtaposition of two aspects or two kinds of pain provides the elements of a quandary which no one wants to recognize. This juxtaposition unveils the vital contradiction with which we are faced. For the negation of pain's functional value belies all of pain's positive claims — as if a witness were proving me guilty of flagrant perjury.

Neither the first claim nor the accusation offers any special food for reflection on the meaning of life. But what astonishes me is the transition, the passage, the reversal from the first face to the second, its about-face (in political terms we would call it a turncoat). How can something suddenly appear as its own opposite? Of course, pain as an enemy would in any case raise the problem of meaning and meaninglessness, but it would inspire in us less revolt if it were only an enemy, if it were frankly itself. Is pain an expression of illness, a signal, or illness itself? Or is it the very face of our adversary, death? If the last were true, then everything would be clear; we would have no reason to argue.

What astonishes us, irritates us, and seems to fuel our resentment (which always flares up against ambivalence, as we know) is that while pain is *this,* it is also *that,* and denies the *this*. While it is *yes,* it is also *no.* (This traitorous yes/no attitude is usually ascribed to the devil.) The important thing is not to see that pain is sometimes useful, sometimes harmful, but to understand by what strange aberration, by what betrayal, having been one, it can become the other. Perhaps this figurative vocabulary of betrayal is shocking, but I have chosen it deliberately, although it lets the underlying resentment show through too clearly not to cast a suspicious light on the dialectic it is meant to express. However, we will see that no other vocabulary would be fitting for the pathos of pain, which is the farthest thing from a cold problem of bookkeeping. Affecting the detachment of a naturalist not only puts me in a position of observing "good manners" where they have no business being observed, but also, and especially, modifies, adulterates, and waters down the very thing that is supposed to stand out — instead of a plate of food, it hands me a menu. For a passionate situation, a passionate vocabulary is required. It is improper for man — for his health, for his honor — to repress his confusion.

If pain, therefore, had not rather insistently shown its purpose, we would have nothing to say. Our only task would be to find a philosophical category for it as a new business adopts a trade name. The situation is more serious because pain has proposed itself officially, scientifically, to fill a function, then has become the object of a court order because of failure to comply. Its new status is lower than that of an annulled statute; it is impossible here to simply mark out with a pen stroke what is engraved in the organism. Its status is lower than an annulment; it is a reversal of signs. Pain goes lower than zero; it is assigned a minus sign. Bankruptcy, collapse, the retreat of a function which denies its own existence, it is not only an evil, but a double evil because of the fact that it was removed, if I may term it thus, from something good!

Functional Pain Replaced by Pathological Pain

Our goal is not to give a detailed description of the different kinds of pain, short or long, tolerable or intolerable, vascular, nervous, or other. For these details other books may be consulted. My desire is to ask three very precise questions.

The first question to be answered by the biologists is: Is there one organ of pain or perhaps more (receivers, channels, centers); and does this organ have a specific function — not merely an incidental recording of painfulness — as an organ of *pain*? Biology's somewhat equivocal answer is: "There are impulse canals which may be severed and illnesses which do attack these channels, such as syringomylia."[1] So there is not a clear organ for pain as there is for seeing or smelling. It is enough, in any case, to be able to deny that we are dealing with pure chance, pure accident, a dispersion at random. We may call it the beginning of an "external purpose." Everything *seems* to indicate that life gave pain a function to perform, that of signaling an approaching or present illness. By an extended figure of speech, we might speak of an *organ* of pain and call it, as I have done, "the organ of illness."

The second question which our biologist is invited to answer is: How is this function accomplished? And the question enables us to unveil the *pseudofinality* of saving pain and reveal it as a pseudoscience stretching from Bernardin de Saint-Pierre's melon[2] to the glorification of pain and trial in the poetry of Alfred de Musset. Pain is my warning signal. Experience is gained because of it: "Man is an apprentice; pain is his master." The problem is that the scientist has trouble controlling his genie in the neutral snares of his measurements, has trouble keeping his head about him. For in point of fact, chronaxies show that pain warns less than it accompanies, orchestrates, amplifies, multiplies, and aggravates the evil. Pain is the blue-tailed fly, an angry bear, superfluous, harmful — the expression of a catastrophe, even more catastrophic in itself. Pain is both a function and the illness of that function, the expression of an illness, and the illness of that expression.

The same agonizing questions keep coming back like a broken record: a function or a catastrophe? An organization? Destructive of organization?

When you think about it, the relation between *pain* and *time* is really closely tied in with the relation between *pain* and *structure*. Does pain have an honest duration, as does any other biological structure with a purpose? Or is its duration only a challenge to the duration of the real biological structures?

[1] Hardly a laughing matter: A terrible disease suppresses what we consider to be the most terrible of evils, pain! A living paradox and an excellent source of reflection: pain legally enthroned, but the absence of pain is thrown out as being illegal! Evil dressed in the garments of virtue, then itself exposed to aggression, to evil! Evil subject to evil. A double function which is equivalent to canceling itself out, to laughing itself to death.

[2] Translator's note: Bernardin de Saint-Pierre was a friend of Jean-Jacques Rousseau and a precursor of romanticism. His firm belief in final causes and providential arrangements led him to assert that the ribs of a melon were designed for its apportionment at the family meal (cf. *The Oxford Companion to French Literature,* p. 64).

This is another way of repeating the same question: Is pain an organization or antiorganization?

I would say, in order to complete our treatment of the relation between pain and time, that the duration of pain is a false one, usurped, just like the duration of any accident which consists of a parasite attacking an independent form. For the form is made to have duration. Pain's duration is only as a challenge and, as it were, as a surprise and a fraud – like someone seizing us by betrayal.

As an antifunction, pain has no legitimate place in time. As we have already emphasized in chapter 2, its existence is only due to its taking up time. Its paradox and its absurdity increase as the usurpation continues.

Pain has no vital consistency of its own. Nevertheless, it manages to occupy a cumbersome place in our lives. *Pain is a parasite of time.* It lives on its substance and impoverishes it to that extent. Time serves no purpose of its own, has no vital role in the accomplishment of pain. Pain simply lives by time, on time.

Time is certainly not an accident of pain, but pain is an accident and a parasite of time.

Pain lives on time, and we have the impression that it lengthens time, prolongs it, feeds on it. An illusion! On the contrary, it empties time instead of filling it out. If times appears to be longer, interminable, while suffering, this is an indefinite, not a definite, phenomenon. It is the opposite of a filling process, which would be filling and shortening of time.

Pain empties time as bleeding empties the body. It leaves time only an empty shell, like a piece of clothing so big that we get lost in it. The indefiniteness of time and pain is a piece of clothing that is much larger because I have shrunk in it; I have been diminished by the very pain I am suffering.

Pain, therefore, gives me a deceptive view of time, and the usurped relation between the two is the farthest thing from essential.

May we conclude, then, that pain is reduced to the level of an unpleasant accident of nature, a breakdown which has compromised its purpose, an anti-nature, an anti-life? Has the organization called life organized its own destruction? Has it provided for, prepared, and orchestrated its own destruction; has it warmed on its own breast the monster which is diminishing it, opposing it, smothering and smashing it? Does meaninglessness have meaning? Does the accident in turn become essence? Is the negation of an organization also an organization? Is disorder order? Are we dealing with a function of catastrophe or with the catastrophe of a function? With a purpose, or an anti-purpose? Does pain express a will for life? Or is this very will opposed, checkmated? The accomplishment of a function or its destruction?

The strange problem of the suffering of a sensitive nerve (a nerve which warns other cells than its own of its suffering) illustrates with a definite example the vicious circle I have been trying to describe and which could too easily be taken as a play on words by a superficial reader. Does the nerve suffer from the pain of the organ which it serves or from its own pain, only provoked by the damaged organ? Does the nerve inform or suffer? Does the pain-carrying nerve receive that pain as the optical nerve receives the sensation of light? — by a *real modification* "concerning which it would be impossible to say," writes Pradines, "whether its effect is to wear out or to maintain." [3] There has been no failure to cite the disconcerting contrast between the nervous centers extremely sensitive to pain, such as the thalamus, and those centers which are themselves completely painless, such as the cerebral cortex, but by which we suffer considerably.

What a paradox! If pain has the function of announcing at the top of its voice the breakdown of a purpose which is life itself, what vicious circle are we led around by its own breakdown? How are we to know when it has itself become threatening? What will be responsible for announcing the disorder of that which is responsible for announcing disorder?

So we see that "sickness-pain" is the sterile negation (in no wise dialectical) of functional pain. Pain as an organ or a function of illness has made a pact with the pain which is itself the illness of that function or that organ. Earlier, I pointed out the absurdity of juxtaposing normal pain and abnormal pain. One is the disavowal of the other. How could we speak of the first, a functional defense mechanism, and then go right on to the second without denying the *raison d'être* of the first and destroying its very meaning as a *normal* function dealing with *abnormal* phenomena? When the *sign* of abnormality is abnormal and we are thus deprived of a *sign*, our whole world is deprived of meaning and floats on a sea of absurdity. Accident-pain, sickness-pain, is the culmination of meaninglessness, because pain was supposed to be the detective combating meaninglessness in the form of accidents and sickness, the watchful guardian of life and meaningfulness. To warn of illness,

[3] Pradines, *Philosophie de la sensation* [The philosophy of sensation], vol. 2, "Les sens de la defense" [The senses of defense], p. 211.

there was supposed to be pain. But what about the illness of pain? Pain communicates and signals meaninglessness to us. But pathological pain unveils the meaninglessness of that definition. If pain is the sign of illness, the illness of that sign consummates its failure as a sign.

Someone will be sure to find that this interpretation of things is far too subtle: *Can not a defense function break down like any other?* This contains the whole mystery of sickness-pain as opposed to "physiological" pain.

It is, in fact, easy to consider things as would a naturalist, as dead objects, juxtaposed, with no meaning for each other. Peter moved his arm. Jack left the room. Nothing communicates the idea of an absurd world better than this purely objective juxtaposition as found in certain modern novels.[4] The same is true if we try to juxtapose pains: The word "and" leaves us ignorant of the fact that these pains carry on between themselves, and with us, living relationships of antagonism and opposition, of which they should be informing us. One or the other: If pain is an accident, an anti-function of nature, how can we explain that nature went to the trouble of endowing it with receivers, channels, and centers to such an extent that it is possible to observe the damage caused by a precise analgesia and to state the rather common opinion that pain is useful? But if, on the contrary, pain has the function we are told it has, we must push to the limit of its consequences the tragic fact that we mobilize all our strength against it. Then Lerich is right and the naturalists are wrong. We must draw all the conclusions, even the absurdity of the kind of care nature put into meticulously preparing this anti-natural monster, this anti-function.

From the viewpoint of anatomy and physiology, everything seems to indicate a rudimentary or aborted organ. But in this case, turning around or deviating from the plan amounts to more than an imperfection. It is an inversion. Pain is an inverted function. Supposed to be a response to evil, it sold itself to evil.

The illness of pain is the worm in the fruit of pain as a function of illness. Pain is a function which bears its own disclaimer. It is not what it is. It lies to what it is. It refuses itself. It is yes and no at the same time: a reflux, a contraction, a resignation. It does away with its own biological meaning; it hides its own absurdity.

[4] On the other extreme, think of the gospel paradox: Jesus spoke in parables *in order that* the people hear without understanding (instead of: *and* the people did not understand).

Harmful pain would be nothing if it were not harmful in just that particular circumstance which it disavows by its useful function. Appearing to be the opposite of what it is in reality is very different from being nothing: a simple accident, a simple lack of meaning. But in this affair the meaning has been spirited away from us.[5] A rape of the meaning is entirely other than the absence of meaning. We have witnessed a falsification. Pain has been altered, denatured — as we say that a mechanism has been falsified, a character perverted, or as a person gives lie to his calling, his promise, or his word.

Pain is not only a valid function which has been inverted or turned around; it is an unfulfilled promise, a lie.

Is it necessary to leave behind biological methods in order to get tangible evidence of such cheating? Yes and no. Yes, as we shall see in the next chapter, if it means leaving science behind in order to ask new questions about data which science satisfied itself with juxtaposing: "There is this kind of pain and then there is this other kind. . . ." No, if one is permitted to be surprised at the contrast between the information coming from one side and that coming from the other. The warning signal of pain is itself disorder; the friend of life is the enemy of life. The biologist only needs a minimum of philosophy (if we can term it thus) to perceive that catastrophic pain disqualifies the anatomical and physiological arguments in favor of pain as an organized structure. The accidents of pain argue in favor of pain as an accident, and against pain as a function. *Of course, the answer will come back that an accident can only result from a valid function,* but here the function meant to warn of accidents ruins itself beyond remedy by appearing as an accident of that function. When the function proper to sickness itself becomes sickness, it commits perjury. It is impossible for pain, by adding pain to pain, to become two and be both the ill form of a function and the functional signal of an illness.

Perversion by Humanization?

How did pain *become* an instinct which devours itself, a vicious circle, biological meaninglessness? How did it become ill?

[5] It is impossible not to take into account this element of deception, of cheating, which removes from the problem of pain any possibility of staying neutral and which transforms it into what we call the "problem of evil." My insistence on repeating this paradox of pain is explained by the singular fact that pain as *evil* has its source there, and nowhere else! This is what I intend to show in this book.

At the beginning it was a part of the real functions of life; it was of service to life. At that time it was not pain, but only a simple defensive reaction. So pain only became pain by ceasing to be itself (that is, a defense reaction)! Pain's painfulness, if you wish, is not within the scope of functional pain, neither is it within the province of the scientist.

How embarrassing! We went out valiantly to conquer a disconcerting reality of life, which is bearing down with all its weight on the human existence, on the world itself. We can legitimately say that around it the entire world is mobilized, centered, concentrated: a central reality, fundamental to human life and civilization. To find it, we went by the serene paths of scientific observation and experimentation and abruptly found the reality we were seeking but with the form of another reality, "of another state of matter," as they say of mutations. It is not the pain for which we were looking, but it is true pain, coming to us, however, by channels other than biological – by our human passion.

On the one hand, this "state" of pain, a mutation, has grown completely out of hand, like a mushroom, losing any proportionality with its initial cause and purpose, deviating and detaching from reality, turning against itself. On the other hand (although it is the same mutation), it duplicates itself with the consciousness and intelligence of pain which is pain itself, which is purely the pain we experience. Growth and consciousness are the two faces of the discontinuity of pain, its conversion, and its monstrous birth.

A mutation just as extraordinary as the appearance of consciousness on the ground of life, pain blends with the consciousness. Human consciousness is a vital lack of meaning. It can turn against itself, turn back up the road of life in the direction whence it came and become an anti-instinct, a refusal – in it we recognize *liberty*. Pain was born with the birth of human liberty.

It seems, therefore, that original pain (a vital reflex partially or completely lacking in painfulness), by becoming the pain by which we are subjected and astonished, lost its first meaning and adopted another in human consciousness. And this conversion is in itself the sum, in one particular aspect of life, of man's *duality*. The dualism of body and consciousness was born of pain,[6] unless this dualism itself is the father of pain.

If this is true, pain lost its role as a bodily function and suddenly

[6] On this point, cf. J. Sarano, *Essai sur la signification du corps,* (Neuchâtel: Delachaux et Niestlé, 1963), chapter 1. English edition is *The Meaning of the Body* (Philadelphia: The Westminster Press, 1966).

became a function of the soul. By its change from one camp to the other, it hastened the division into two separate camps. It is largely responsible for the appearance and fossilization of a *dualism of body and soul.* In any case, pain is no longer to be found in the biologists' camp, but in the spiritual world. Its metaphysical importance has increased. By becoming human, it became metaphysical.

It could only become properly *pain* by escaping the realm of biology, by escaping the gravity of science, by thus furnishing the proof of its irreducibility to any approach of a scientific nature. Henceforth it is beyond such a scope. Pain is not pain, is not painful except by its mockery of any scientific maneuver. By its conversion into a disease of man's consciousness, it is irretrievably beyond the grasp of science. This illness, this inadaptation to life grafted onto a vital adaptation, requires and proves its need of something else, a plan of research other than biological explanation, a plan of research of a spiritual nature.

The Irreducible Nature of Painfulness

You may be asking why the warping of a phenomenon should remove it from the province of science. Is it no longer a phenomenon, no longer an object to be studied and explained, no longer an object of observation and experimentation? Even if it has become absurd and dangerous, a valid function still belongs to its family; it is impossible for it to disown its ancestors; it is still homogeneous with itself.

This is doubtlessly true. But here we are dealing with something entirely different. For by becoming painful, pain was no longer homogeneous with itself. Biology may explain how it took a wrong turn as far as the effectiveness of its defensive signals is concerned, but it can never explain why pain is—*painful.*

Let us suppose that, at the very best, a scientist were able to answer affirmatively these two questions which we have already studied: (1) Did nature give pain a role to play? Yes. (2) Is it accomplishing its function? Perfectly. There would still be *a third question,* which it is absolutely impossible for a scientist to answer: (3) If this role is being correctly fulfilled (or incorrectly—that has no importance for this point), what is its relationship with the *sui generis* quality of the painfulness of pain? Why does this function, even if it is accomplished, include painfulness? Is painfulness indispensable for pain?

The painful quality of pain is not self-evident, and this is a bit of delicate ground which I must explore. But my undertaking seems to have been compromised from the very beginning. How is it possible to propose seriously to separate pain from pain? The passage from an observation of fact to a rightful necessity is automatic. But how can we speak of right in this area? *That's the way it is,* and that's that. And, to be courteous, one adds, if a harm-inducing stimulus did not induce *pain,* how would we know to *avoid* it? A reaction of repulsion and flight when faced with a nociceptive stimulus necessarily *implies* the unpleasant quality (which we call *pain* in its widest sense) of the nociceptive experience.

The argument seems obvious at first sight. However, for those who are willing to hear me out, there will be no difficulty in distinguishing repulsion (a *behavioral* term) and pain (a term denoting *sensation*). I will call to mind once again the distinction which Pradines emphasizes between "the motorial aversion which is of a rather adaptive nature: its ordinary effect is to avert a harmful agent," and "the consciousness of pain which accompanies it . . . and which it is impossible to include as a part of its adaptive nature." [7]

When we repeat the old saw that if the experience were not painful, we would go to no trouble to avoid it, we forget that the negative behavior (of flight) with respect to the nociceptive stimulus does not necessarily imply the distressing (painful) nature of the experience.

It is not difficult to give factual proof:

1. It is well known that the retreat or flight of a living body attacked by a nociceptive stimulus *precedes* what may properly be called pain and, as it were, anticipates it. Conclusion: *Pain was never needed.* The slower conduction times of the pain fibers enable us to put our finger on the dissociation of which I am speaking. Defense can therefore be conducted without any real pain, since the former takes place *before* the latter.

[7] "There is no reason why this (the consciousness of pain) should ameliorate reflexes, since it adds to them no knowledge of the evil involved and apparently only tacks on pain itself. Pain can be an error or an anomaly of nature, without the reflex of aversion being one. Let us go on to the defects which this reflex has inherited from pain. The blame we can level at it is its ignorance and distraction; it reacts to minute evils and does not respond to serious diseases; it does not always orient its defense measures toward those points which are really in danger. It is clear that pain has rescued it from none of these insufficiencies. But it would not be a good description of pain's misdeeds to limit the evil it accomplishes to the insufficiencies of the reflex action. The evil of pain is pain itself" (Pradines, *op. cit.,* pp. 129–130). It would be difficult to identify better the two levels at which the problem of pain arises.

Experiments carried out both on inferior animals and on higher mammals under anesthesia (or with the brain removed) show the same obvious, tangible separation between behavior-of-pain and pain itself. We have emphasized enough that the art of experimentation has, by working with subjects proper to its methods, deprived us of what we are dealing with, of pain itself. But at least it has the useful side effect of making obvious the discrimination between *motor aversion* and *pain.*

2. The preceding argument is sufficient alone, and I would like to add here a few reflections on the same theme.

Does the struggle for life, natural selection, and vital competition necessarily entail pain? Is it possible to put pain on the level of an indispensable principle of life?

For if the living being is defined as the expansion of a center of individuation and of duration, which creates its own environment, which traces out its own territory, choosing, selecting, rejecting or assimilating, destroying or incorporating, following the criteria of harmfulness or usefulness, if it makes its own way by ruthlessly orienting the universe according to its need of creating and recreating itself, is it not inevitable, then, that anything not of service to it risks rendering a disservice.

Not at all, and for two complementary reasons. First, because selection in no way implies the necessity of aversion or threat, the choice may be made between what is *useful* and what is *indifferent.* There is no need for the choice to be made between what is useful and what is dangerous. The choice may be made without, in turn, becoming harmful, without impeding the choices to be made by other living beings. Neither does selection imply Darwinian *selection* which implies competition. *Competition* is not included in the selection and assimilation necessary for the conservation of life. The existence of mortal *competition* is absolutely original; one must eat one's neighbor and in turn be eaten.[8] This is an evil

[8] Conservation and perpetuation of life, instead of being helped by pain (on the individual level), are carried out by the wasteful means of reproduction on the level of the species. Individuals are swallowed and massacred by the thousand. Nature has made hardly any provision for the individual's defense, in spite of what the organ of pain may have led us to think. The pain of being devoured by a wild beast is no guarantee, as far as I can tell, that the first experience will keep a second of its kind from happening again. A bird's terror of a carnivore does not keep it from being one day eaten. It is even ridiculous; terror often leads, not to flight, but to paralyzed immobility, fascination, passivity, and defenselessness! The horrible designs of nature! Does it not in truth seem more as though, instead of organizing the defense of living beings, it were putting its genius to organizing and amplifying useless pain, dangerous pain, disastrous pain?

irreducible to any other consideration and inherent in selective needs and selective love as much as in defense. They are closely associated. Love is a defense of the species. Love, conquest, danger, struggle, fear, and death are all part of the same tragedy of life. But this tragedy, in which the role of pain is easily perceived, could have gotten along without pain, both because selection does not imply competition, and because competition, although it may imply motor aversion, does not imply pain. *Evil,* an alien problem (or mystery), here appears in its naked reality.

3. From arguments of *fact* I have passed to arguments of *justice.* When I said, *"could have gotten along without pain,"* is this not encroaching on the unfathomable sources and ends of Creation? What right do we have to extrapolate beyond what is?

In reality, the mental operation of "imagining" a defense function deprived of pain has no more interest than experimenting with Bacon's method of variations. The operation effects mentally the dissociation which experimentation and life itself have operated in *fact.* Its final purpose would be to show that from a connection established *in fact,* we have no reason to conclude that there is a necessary connection established *in justice.*

The warning of danger and pain are by no means connected by right, although they often are in fact. We must not consider a frequent connection, or even a *constant* one, to be *necessary.*

The *sui generis* nature of pain (as a function), of being *painful,* is by no means implied in its role (if we suppose it is being fulfilled) as an alarm signal serving the living being. *That is how it is in fact,* so much so that it has seemed inevitable that we must learn to avoid danger by the pain it causes.[9]

But *by right, "things should have come about otherwise."* This phrase is no gratuitous game of our imagination, nor does it translate some resentment harbored against things as they now stand.[10] It expresses the dissociation between the facts and the right, between constancy and necessity. "Things should have come about otherwise": The organ of every-man-for-himself, of defense and flight, could very well have used a means just as prompt (comparable to sight or the sexual instinct),[11] just as effective and

[9] Congenital indifference to pain, for example, ceases to be truly dangerous, thanks to education, which advantageously replaces the harmful experience.

[10] The commonsense remark "Accept things as they are" has no theoretical worth and could never satisfy the problem we have before us here.

[11] Let us recall that the fibers of pain have a conduction time which is slower than the fibers of touch, for example. That is a strange thing for the messengers of vital danger.

specific, but which would have caused no suffering to the person.

The painfulness of pain is not summed up in its function as a signal or an expression,[12] nor in the notion of danger or motor aversion. Pain as a vital or natural necessity is a false notion.

4. Another way of expressing the irreducibility of painfulness is in its description as an experience just as original, *sui generis,* "absurd," as is the sweetness of sugar or the color red. I will end with this point for it marks the line of demarkation between the possibilities offered by science and those offered by philosophy for understanding pain.

The fact that pain exercises this function of a negative tropism in response to danger, by aversion and flight, no more implies that it should be painful than that it should be green or salty. Nausea, bitterness, and bad odors seem to be so tied in with the sensation that they blend together. Nevertheless, unpleasantness is not the sensation itself; neither is the pleasure which the sensation may cause to be confused with the sensation itself. Green may be unpleasant to me, but its unpleasantness is not to be confused with its greenness. We lack the vocabulary to designate distinctly a given odor and the unpleasant repulsion with which it is associated for us. We do know, however, that excrements charm the senses of insects and birds. For them the smell of roses emanates from a manure pile. As they say, "There is no accounting for tastes. . . ."

The *sui generis* experience of pain is unexplainable, and especially is it unexplainable by scientific means. The most precise measurements can never justify green's being green, nor can they show, by proving identical wave lengths, that your green is mine.

The presence or the absence of the quality of pain has no effect on science. It is a blind point over which the most detailed of studies will have no power. For painfulness is *of an order different* from the pain with which they deal. Judge from this hypothetical situation: Imagine that functional pain is given a form entirely different from what we call "painfulness" (unpleasantness or oppressiveness). *The scientist would not even perceive its presence.* The presence or absence of painfulness has no effect on the scientist's operations. If you ask him if pain as a sensation is a condition *sine qua non* of functional pain, he will not understand what you are talking about. Or if he does understand and answers, it is be-

[12] We do not consider signal and expression to be the same thing, but it is impossible for an expression to be a catastrophic reaction, just as absurd as an emotion which paralyzes without also being intentional. We believe that pain is expression/sign, with the two elements indissolubly linked.

cause he is a man who has suffered pain. A structure or a function has in itself, because it is what it is, no color or savor.

The scientist can decide questions of the type which we asked in the preceding chapters: Is there a function, an organ which responds to what we call a sensation of pain? (Just as we would ask: What is the organ corresponding to the sensation of sight?) Does this organ accomplish its function? In short, then, although science may show that pain is a response to imperative demands for the defense and conservation of the organism, it can never tell us *why this function is "painful."* Science literally does not know what this means.

When science talks about pain, it is talking about everything except pain. And we have every right to ask ourselves if the problem with which we are dealing is not radically foreign to biology. The quality of the *painful* experience concerns the *subject.* It is beyond the realm of science since the vocation of the latter is objectivity, since it deals only with *objects.* When the problem of pain is closely analyzed, it is seen to concern philosophy, that is, questioning the meaning of creation. It is a philosophical problem and may be considered in no other way.

5

One Failure—Master over Two Domains: At the Origin of the Problem of Evil

We now understand the urgent necessity of changing our plan of attack. Pain – to the extent that it is *painful* – is incapable of domestication, of reduction to a mere biological equation with some psychological and sociological implications. In its "irreducibility" pain shows up both the insufficiency of *natural* data and the reasons for searching elsewhere. It is both a scandal and a stimulant, vexation and appeal. The scientist objectively demands of pain its justification, and when he gets none, he is forced to "pass," to use card-playing terms. Pain brings out both the requirements and the limits of the scientist. With the same movement pain is rejected and respected. The scientist rightfully demands an account, but at the same time renounces any answer, and recognizes that it is someone else's job to make this demand. Whatever progress science may make in explaining the mechanism of pain, it will *still* be true, and will always be true, that the mechanism cannot explain the essential point: the painfulness of pain. This function may show itself to be essential, but that is not an explanation of the essential nature of the function: not just provoking defense reactions, but *also* being painful.

At the beginning of this book I wrote that it is possible to furnish two types of explanations of pain: as a defense system for the organism and by original sin – by the complicated channels of the nervous system or by the channels (no less complicated in men's eyes) of the divine economy.

The prestige of the first type of explanation, which we may call scientific, is due to its foundation in experimentation, what we call "experimental data." But if science describes, no matter how minutely, the nerve endings for the reception of pain, conducting channels, centers, mechanisms, and even a coarse finality, inaccurate and faulty, this explanation still leaves us desirous of more. For neither anatomy nor physiology, experimentation, psychology, sociology, nor any other science of objective facts will ever explain the irreducibility of pain to objective data. None of these data will ever explain the *painful* nature of this strange function of the living being.

Drawing from less positive sources, from philosophical reflection and the "assertions without proof" of faith, the other type of explanation has, nevertheless, the decisive advantage of answering directly our questions about pain: Why pain? Why is pain painful? This second type of explanation is no longer only an explanation; it is something else. At the first try it meets our ultimate requirements of justification, comprehension, and meaning.

Rare are the explanations which are equivalent to a comprehension. When a scientist tells us the *how* of a laboratory dissection, he unveils nothing about the *why*. He does not go beyond the organs he is observing. When the biblical author tells us "how things happen," to take an example on the opposite extreme, he immediately gets down to the "why": "Why do we suffer?" [1]

When the philosopher or the believer claims, for example, that pain is a part of "God's plans" (for our mistakes, for our salvation, etc.), he is speaking of *pain* and not of some function with which pain has accidentally, pathologically, and nonessentially become associated. As I have said, if you take the pain out of pain, the scientist's explanation will stay the same down to the last letter, the last comma. He didn't even notice it was gone! But if you take the painfulness out of pain, the philosophical explanation vanishes; there is nothing more to explain. This is why we were wrong when we first knocked on the scientist's laboratory door. We were not talking about the same thing, but to our own confusion we were using the same word.

Philosophical Status and Biological Status Do Not Mix

What began as a scientific problem, as the nerves, channels, centers, and behavior of pain prove (and I insist on this point), must nevertheless be abandoned by the scientist as out of his field.

Then the philosopher (in the widest sense of the term) steps up, strong in his advantage over the first contestant, armed with well-polished arguments: "We must consider the partiality of our view-

[1] Of course, I am not saying that myth is enough to satisfy the rationalist or even the true believer. No one in this latter category is satisfied with taking the story of original sin *literally*, nor will he consider original sin to be a sufficient justification for the world's evil. More on this later.

points as finite creatures," he intones. "We who are so ignorant of the cosmic or divine economy — all this must be very closely examined!" As though he were the first to study pain! But such is not the case. We have seen only too much of the evidence on pain. Things are not explained so easily, and pain has a singularly "loaded past." The philosopher must sooner or later realize that the scientist has quite involuntarily made his task very difficult. The metaphysical "virtues" of pain could get along quite well without its biological virtues; they could, in fact, get along a thousand times better with a pain without biological pretentions — and especially without overpraised pretension.

The philosophical status of pain has not finished suffering from its biological next-door neighbor.

In other circumstances the philosophical explanation takes over for the scientific with no problem. One, for example, defines man in terms of the monkey, the other by his mind, without the second feeling that it has been cruelly belied by the first. The notion of a monkey *that has made it* does not absolutely clash with the notion of a supernatural calling.

But the case of pain is entirely different. Philosophy does not have the task of investing a pain that has succeeded with a metaphysical ministry — far from it. It is not dealing with pain, *but with the failure of pain,* with its lamentable biological *fiasco,* with the betrayal which made of it an enemy of the being it was supposed to serve.

Judge for yourself: If pain were what it is — an organ and a function of life — if it were succeeding in that for which it seems biologically to be made, *there would be no place for a philosophy of pain.*

Considering the two types of explanation which I mentioned, it becomes clear that it would be unintelligent to judge them one after the other, one without the other. They must be taken and judged *by each other.* Neither of the two can cancel out the existence of the other. Philosophical reflection especially cannot ignore the other, as one tries to discredit a bothersome witness. It is indispensable for the philosopher, before linking the problem of pain with the problem of evil, to reflect on what this connection of the two problems *presupposes,* on the tremendous avowal implied by the fact alone that we are now speaking of the "problem of evil." And we must become acutely aware of this avowal: *Pain is an evil;* that is, made for one function, it missed its calling and is henceforth a falsehood against life.

Philosophical status appears, therefore, both as a requirement of mankind and an adventure with no escape, or at least one that is extremely hazardous. Is the philosophical status of pain compatible with the wrecked biological status of pain? It is too late now to shut the door and call it a simple failure; the *evil* has been done!

The question then is not only to know if each of these two types of explanation is sufficient or insufficient, nor is it to know which is the most insufficient! The issue is rather to examine seriously whether these two modes (both of which we are obliged to notice; the most bothersome of which we cannot ignore or destroy) – whether these two groups of evidence – can coexist peaceably; whether one is the ruin of the other; whether one hastens the bankruptcy of the other; or whether they are mutually harmful, instead of supporting and completing each other.

The two impasses of pain: What are they?

1. The biological evidence is an appeal to open up another type of evidence. Pain has no biological *meaning;* it is a foreign language, an incomprehensible absolute, an absolute unknown, absolute meaninglessness. Unsalvaged pain, not understood by the scientist, stays on like a foreign body in our experience, a scandal, an evil. It is therefore an appeal to open up new evidence, an appeal which is only the impasse of the first method of investigation. Another means of locomotion must be taken to pass this difficult ford.

Having braked to a stop in this dead end, it might be useful to remind the one who has spoken of pain, and is now speaking of evil, that he has changed levels – that is obvious – but also that this change is an avowal of capital importance. It is the changeover which is important. Discussions on this new plane, progressively reducing pain to our level and understanding it, are something else. And before we can get around to doing that, we have to pronounce this word and pose its problem – a word whose brevity is inversely proportional to its enormous importance. Pronouncing it means establishing it on a certain level, means ratifying and consummating the absurdity of pain on the level of our biopsychological life. The changeover is therefore of utmost importance, one of the keys to our study.

2. But, unfortunately, there is another impasse. Not only does the very fact of establishing the philosophical status mean accepting its vital failure, whether implicitly and consciously or not, *but that very failure makes very difficult the task of the one who is trying to take over and assemble the evidence for the philosophical*

case. This is another essential point of change, another narrow passage (in speleological terms), in which we are stuck right now.

The Problem Child of Science,
The Spoiled Child of Philosopher and Believer

It is only with a full knowledge of the facts that the philosopher must take up the burden of pain. But not without effort will he be able to make a fallen biological instrument into an instrument of the spirit.

A defensive reaction, an expression and an alarm signal, useful for the conversation of the living organism – experience shows it to be entirely different, the reversal, the contradiction of what it had announced, the enemy of life; and then they whisper in our ear that it is a life-giving obstacle. When it fulfills its role, they say nothing. But when it fails, they say it is a trial to be fought through, to be overcome, to be accepted for our elevation.

The logical conclusion would be that the misfortune of betraying a function is a means of obtaining special merit.

Too often we try to make both sides work. Pain cannot play *both* roles when they are the opposite of each other. It cannot be both *biological* (an alarm signal in the service of life) and, when it turns against life, *spiritual* (a more or less mysterious trial).

It is impossible to put pain to work in a spiritual field just because it failed its biological function, nor can one make an insufficiency into a virtue.

As an example, it would be nothing spiritually to insert pain into the divine plan if that were not the disavowal of what must also be legitimately called part of the divine plan: pain as a defense organ of the living creature. Its spiritual office must necessarily be built on the shattered pieces of its former function; it is made of its defeat. Thus the spiritual "plan" turns the biological plan to derision, and such a double usage destroys the very notion of a "plan."

This is why it seems indispensable to me to *confront,* not only to justify, the two types of explanations which I have mentioned. Pulling him by the coat sleeve as though to bring him back to earth, I would whisper into the ear of the philosopher who would prove too much: "Don't forget that the pain you have inherited has already served elsewhere, and your beautiful discourses cannot pretend to be unaware of that fact. Don't forget the humble and suspicious origins of pain. It only succeeds so well with you because – poor student that it is – it failed elsewhere!"

By what sleight of hand can the philosopher transform a lost cause into a spiritual office for pain? What miracle can make the problem child of science into the spoiled child of the metaphysician and believer? Trial, heroism, courage? How nice! Sin, redemption? Wonderful!

Yes, don't forget the humble and suspicious origins of pain. Under the respectable name of "the problem of evil," pain becomes a philosophical personage. It was necessary to begin by unmasking the usurper, to show the doubtful beginnings of this great bastard lord, the result of a mistake in life!

Part 2
Suffering as Mediation

1

The Importance of Implications

"Thus pain is only the consciousness of being pain; it is that state the perception of which causes conscious suffering." [1]

Our study of pain has led us to the recognition of the existence of evil in this world. One does not know everything nor does one say everything there is to say about a subject of reflection. What is said does not suffer from what is not said as long as the reader is forewarned. Suffering is an experience which may be confronted from many sides and in every way. My viewpoint will not be, is incapable of being, theological. Certain questions which the theologian must confront will not detain me here. Not, of course, that I consider them any less legitimate. Those which I will attack seem, for the time being at least, to be most apt to lead me to the center of the mystery. Perhaps the theological approach will suit someone other than myself. My goal is not a *summa theologica,* but a personal itinerary.

The Constitution of Evil

As always, my first appeal will be to get down to the "things" in question, to forget all "knowledge" of this subject which extends beyond the realm of human history, which is contained in some ready-made theory. This approach is what some will call an "objective spirit." Our *modus vivendi* with pain, with evil itself, must be worked out by each of us, each in his own way. "Ordinarily," wrote Pascal, "we persuade ourselves better with the reasons we have found ourselves." But the same path should be adoptable by others. My considerations should be usable for a journey in common.

[1] Maurice Blondel, *L'Action* (Paris: Presses Universitaires de France, 1893), p. 455.

What will getting down to the things in question mean in this case? This plan may be more ambiguous than it seems. It will make itself the subject of my reflections.

To confront evil *directly,* to take away the habitual screen of explanations — is such a thing possible? My first observation on this point must be that observation is an abstraction, a pure illusion. We approach this idea of evil with a burden of years, of cultural attitudes, of moral and religious meanings — all built up around a word which we thought to be simple.

Evil cannot be reduced to an immediate fact. *It is an experience.* And if someone wants to exhaust this experience, to live out and extract the pure objective essence of evil — which would make it independent of our individual, social, and human manner of life — if someone wants to make it his own, the operation will be illusory and especially dangerous because of the very thing he was trying to isolate.

For this reality is only a reality as long as it refuses to be isolated and as long as no one has isolated it. We must beware of analysis and only make use of it while keeping in mind that it is but an operation and that its results are only the results of analysis.

Evil designates in a nutshell everything "that doesn't go right" in this world. We feel it in our pains and in those of other creatures, in our failures, our illnesses, our hates, our faults — in every wrong that we *commit* and in every trial we *go through.* And it is difficult for us to perceive clearly the relationship between the classes of evil as separated by philosophers: moral evil and metaphysical evil.

There is a classic method of "treating" evil: define it, show of what it consists, try to find a justification for it, and as it were, assign "responsibilities" — a fallaciously "objective" method. In their study of the "mystery" of evil, several philosophers, led by Gabriel Marcel, have concluded that this strange problem is not a problem, in the sense "that it encroaches on its own data, that it takes them over and thereby oversteps its role as a simple problem." [2]

I would prefer to think of the question in this form: What is necessary for the problem of evil to arise? What are the conditions that make the problem possible? What is implied by such a problem?

Methods of approach, preliminaries, presuppositions, environments, conditioning factors, and conditions — all these seem to

[2] G. Marcel, *Le monde cassé* [The broken world], p. 267.

me in their own way more important than the habitual explanations and refutations.

The seed of the solution to a problem may already be found in the choice of method. There are fewer means of solving a problem, if you wish, than there are ways of posing it. And the solution is contained in the way the problem is attacked.

Such a fact here takes on particular significance. We must say that my *personal* response expresses the sum of my life experience, and the sole fact that I have selected this problem, have halted to study it, am speaking of "evil," is already an expression and an unveiling of myself. But even more, *man in general* being able to *speak* of "evil," to stop and look at this problem (as a projector can stop the action of a film) and to isolate it under the name "evil," bears witness to the humanity of a certain manner of dealing with things which we must elucidate.

In short, such a debate must begin by "psychoanalysis." What are the reasons, open or secret, conscious or unconscious, for *my* predilection for such a bothersome quest? What is the condition of the human consciousness or subconscious *in general,* and what is the condition of the human mind, of human logic, which will make possible a quest into evil, which will enable *the notion itself* of evil to make its way into the human consciousness and finally into the language?

Using a vocabulary in vogue, we might say that if it did not have a particular kind of "intentionality," "evil" would not have been able to carve out a niche in the compact mass of reality. And it might be said, using the same vocabulary, that there is a problem of the *constitution* of evil considered as a problem or as a notion — constitution with its Husserlian meaning, so ambiguous, of an unveiling which creates (or constitutes).

Our clearest task is to conduct an inquiry into the origins of the idea of evil and the ups and downs of the human pathway implied by those origins. More than just a point of departure, this problem is rapidly transformed into the terminal, the point of arrival. No longer is it self-evident; now it appears complex, heavy with individual history and with the history of mankind. But this history has nothing to do with the history of the treatments the problem has received through the years. This experiential history is rather hidden under the surface, implicit, just as manifest in what is not said as in explicit history based on reason and fact. It is the bearer of an anthropology of evil, a cosmology, a theology, a prolegomena to evil.

But if we must take evil from behind, by its sudden motives, we must do so without forgetting our "practical" viewpoint. Whatever reproaches may be brought against the uselessness of these problems, life backs us up against the wall too often for us to scorn them. Several years ago I began otherwise a note on evil: "Morals are an expression of man's effort to adapt himself to the alien existence of evil in the world. One cannot be understood without the other. Evil exists; let us be frank enough to look it in the eye. Then we can ask ourselves what our attitude will be toward it, what our morality will be. . . ."

Would I today speak in the same fashion? Looking evil in the eye cannot be done unequivocally. It is an abstraction to believe that morals could be an after-response to evil, like one actor following another onto the stage. May we insist: Speaking of evil, posing the problem, is making it into a thing. The terms themselves presuppose civilization, morality, and religion (even within unbelief). It is artificial to say that evil and morals originate in each other. One is the other. Although my morality, my concrete conduct in life, neither follows nor precedes "my solution to the problem of evil," it is at least an expression of the response which consciously or unconsciously, explicitly or not, I have given to that problem. And it is impossible to deny that "evil is man." (It defines man's outlook, the turn of his mind as a man.

This evil bears witness to man, both in his individuality and in his humanity.

The most theoretical problems, apparently the idlest ones, nevertheless bear their *testimony*. They have practical worth, pedagogical worth, worth for life. They help to situate us in the concreteness of life, its urgency, its day-to-dayness. Evil expresses what we are; it contributes its part in making us what we are — by its very expression.

It is therefore useful for me to ask myself — for us to ask ourselves — this question, a question which must be more untiringly asked and re-asked than any other: Do pain and evil require a theory or a practical response? Or a response which is a theory (a praxis)? A knowing and an acting at the same time? It has been said that whatever it may cost us, since we have to confront it, it is better to face pain with a proper reaction than with good arguments. But every argument bears witness to a behavior, and such a dichotomy hides the unity of theory and of life.

I was saying that speaking of "evil" is not only setting up the problem; in a certain sense it is already giving it a solution. Before appearing as a quest, the word "evil" is a response. Included, enveloped within itself, it contains the response which we must explain and unfold. For our knowledge of evil is not an objective knowledge. I myself am implied in it. An "evil" which is the object of pure observation would only be an observational illusion. Writing elsewhere I once said that a pretension to cold objectivity is the most subjective of illusions.[3] Of course, some may consider this implication of the entire man in the problem of evil as a *contaminated* adhesion – to be psychoanalytically peeled of its questionable motivations. I rather believe that this *contamination, which is due to our human flesh, is a part of the very thing we are studying and that it would be destroying the nature of evil to take away its flesh.*

Someone will be sure to answer that I have gotten nowhere by this confusion of evil and flesh. Must the *fact* not be distinguished from my judgment, from my attitude in the face of this *fact*? "Evil is a fact," writes R. Verneaux, "a datum of experience." [4] So call this datum, this fact, "evil" and add that the way we utilize this fact depends on us. Nothing could be clearer than that.

My purpose is to ask if a datum called "evil" is warrantable or if "evil" is not rather of such a nature as to be "evil" only when we have "utilized" it. The utilization to which I put evil already contains my answer, and later I will be able to state that evil *is* its own condemnation. Such a viewpoint would keep us from provoking the seductive precept that evil becomes or produces good thanks to the use that I (or God) have made of it.[5]

How are we to explain the asceticism of those men who speak of evil as an *evil,* but still accept it, assume it while at the same time condemning it? We must, in fact, emphasize the nuance between evil in its *meaning for all of humanity* and evil as it is loaded

[3] Jacques Sarano, *Médecine et médecins* [Medicine and physicians] (Paris: Editions du Seuil, 1959), p. 92.

[4] R. Vernaux, *Problèmes et mystères du mal* [Problems and mysteries of evil] (Paris: Editions de La Colombe, 1956), p. 35.

[5] "The devil himself carries his stone." For Claudel, evil is "like a slave who hauls up the water" *(Repos du 7e jour* [Seventh day rest], Act III). Fenelon: "God has often promised that the heathen would further his plans by their crimes" (Francois Fénelon, *Oeuvres,* Editions de Paris, vol. 4, p. 10). And Malebranche: "God uses the heathen even to carry out his plans, but disorder is still just that" (Third Reply to the First Book of *Réflexions* by M. Arnaud) quoted by P. de Lubac, *La pensée religieuse du P. Teilhard de Chardin* [The religious thought of Father Teilhard de Chardin] (Paris: Aubier Montaigne), p. 152.

on each of our shoulders according to our attitudes and personal strengths. Of course, it is impossible to have good practices and bad theories on evil. But it is possible to have a good philosophy in act and a bad philosophy in word if we follow the words we have learned, which categorize a *thing* called evil like a broken animal which we are supposed to have tamed.

We must be careful here not to give evil the value of an hypostasis; it must appear in the mixed reality of its man/world nature. Some would call it the schema for a mode of operation.[6]

Evil is other than itself: I mean by this that it is outside the scope of a fact, a thing, a datum. It contains more than a thing. Not only does it imply all our individual, cultural, and historical presuppositions, but also the objectifying attitude which tries to situate evil as evil and thereby finally denies it, goes beyond it, and transcends it with the same movement as that which "constituted" it as evil.

Neutralizing Evil, a Nonexistent Problem

Before dealing with evil as a thing, therefore, we must give our attention to that act which isolates it and constitutes it isolatedly as a thing, a reality. Perhaps we would be helped in this quest by an inventory of the conditions for the *absence* of evil. The agenesis or the atrophy, if I may use such terms, of evil as a thing would illuminate this evil just as an incurable disease makes healing stand out more clearly.

What is the reality of evil for an animal, the humble man *subject* (in the strongest sense of the term) to evil, the pleasure-seeker who for a moment forgets it or fears it without knowing his own thoughts, the believer without a fault in his armor who wipes it out with his first blow, or, finally, the man of action in the heat of battle? Is evil only a halt in the direct confrontation of life? Is it proper and right to get out of the main stream of life in order to objectify, to *name* evil, and thus to make oneself an accomplice of the notion of evil?

[6] Modern phenomenology refuses to imagine the abstraction of a fact or a world deprived of human consideration or praxis. "It would be prudent to make of no schema an hypostasis" (H. Duméry, *Philosophie de la religion* [The philosophy of religion], vol. 1, p. 80; cf. Merleau-Ponty, *Phénoménologie de la perception* [The phenomenology of perception], p. 494. (English translation of Duméry's book is *The Problem of God in the Philosophy of Religion,* trans. Courtney, (Evanston: Northwestern University Press, 1964); that of Merleau-Ponty's book: *Phenomenology of Perception,* trans., C. Smith, (New York: Humanities Press, Inc., 1962).

A pantheism in love with totality would refuse to remove itself from its cosmic solidarity and would contest our right to stop the projector on one frame and then call that picture evil. We would meet with the same indignation in our technical civilization from the militant partisans of struggle and love. Evil, they tell us, is a *nonexistent problem.* There are only concrete problems, in the plural, for which particular solutions must be proposed. Every partial difficulty serves as an obstacle and as a base for an effective series of victories. Evil *does not exist.* This statement is less than an opinion of the world; we can discern in it the sign of a negative attitude, a weakness – passing or durable, individual or collective – just as death "is a civilian idea" for a fighting soldier.[7]

In short, according to this view, speaking of "evil" is not setting up a problem; it is a failure to meet the problems raised by life.

The believer will speak in other terms, but will come to the same conclusion. Speaking of "evil," is it not refusing to give to the Creator the credit due for his love? Criticism is improper; cooperation is what counts. It is up to us to make the world into something better. By our *liberty* the "problem" will take on another form. Whether or not there is a "problem of evil" depends, in the end, on us.[8]

The pluralistic pragmatism of the first approach and the cooperative spirit of the second have a certain amount of truth, and I just might be in agreement with them: but *afterwards* (this is essential and sums up my approach in one word)! Let us not mistake a settled problem for the absence of a problem! An "activist" solution (in its best sense) has cut right through the scandalous knot and run right through what was supposed to be a moment's halt before objectified evil. Its success is nevertheless secondary: It is a result, the exile's return to a reconciliation which it would like to be initial, but which must not be confused with the real initial situation (the pre-critical situation).

It is enough for the question of evil to have been asked *once* in the universe, for it to be here before us, alien, insolent; and nothing can erase the fact that the problem has been posed and recog-

[7] P. Voivenel, *Le médecin devant la douleur et la mort* [The physician and his encounter with pain and death], quoted by P. L. Landsberg, *Essai sur l'expérience de la mort* [A study on the experience of death] (Paris: Editions du Seuil), p. 40.

[8] To this aspect of faith we should add the two themes of incomprehensible (incommensurable) divinity on the one hand, and freedom in sin, on the other (see next chapter). Here I am only calling to mind those problems which obstruct the question at its inception, at its departure.

nized. Would refusing to recognize the problem not be the act itself of recognizing it? Would it not be giving it an answer without agreeing to do so? Contesting the legitimacy of the problem is answering while refusing to answer. We might just as well act out in the open. Perhaps we will come back to that cooperation with creation, but *after* having agreed to confront the scandal as it stands.

If we can take it, reflection on the problem of evil can be only healthy; it can only give meaning to our lives. It is a question worth struggling with, worth the test it brings to bear on us, worth the trouble. What would we win by pretending not to see it, by camouflaging our solutions as so-called "worthless questions"? If solutions are presented as solutions, their value as victories will be all the greater. In my opinion, the game of "nonexistent problems" is often a poor game, "a bad quarrel." It goes around difficulties, haughtily turns away from them. On the other hand, it is good warfare (and in good faith) to respect those who groan at the thought of questioning evil, even if it is with the puerile vociferations of impenitent rationalism or a wordy battle of sharpened arguments. It is proper to enter into someone else's thoughts even if we think somewhat conceitedly that he is far behind us. We have been through all that; we know there is no use acting tough. It would be better for us to get back together again after the dialogue, better to meet on the basis of a common evolution which will not be a repudiation but a transformation. There is no such thing as getting along without a process of maturation; I know from my own costly experience. Now I am less tempted than I used to be to think myself ahead of the pack.

Evil, Irreducible Reality

Is not the "absence" of evil simply being afraid to look at it? Does not evil fill the whole horizon with its brutal omnipresence? How could we turn our eyes from this evil — the limit of reality, original, present before any question can be asked — before any reaction can take place to that presence, irreducibility itself? Who can conjure away the tragic reality of a child or of an animal in pain, even before that pain bears the name of evil (or when it only bears the name because of my presence)?

The extent of this primary suffering is as vast as the oceans, inexhaustible. And it is even more fearful because it is inaccessible to the conscience, to words, or to the senses. Blind, deaf, wide open, it offers its defenseless breast without retreat, without possibility of restoration in some attitude, some justification, some philosophy, or some belief.

This raw evil, nameless, faceless, this evil which has not yet been circumscribed, domesticated, exorcised, dominated by a name; this pain which has not yet been formulated, which does not even know that it is pain, tied and gagged into solitude, buried in itself, and all the more disarmed and vulnerable for all that – this evil and this pain appear to my eyes as unjustifiable in the extreme, what we might call absolute evil. For no explanation can lighten the crushing weight of this pain suffered in all its force. By no consolation is it appeased, from the most comprehensive answers to those most revolting by their lack of philosophical or doctrinal finesse. It stands out then and always as a reproach to the universe, an inextinguishable thirst for justice which nothing can satisfy.

The irreducible reality of naked pain stands up like an obsession in the line of fire of whoever decides to speak of evil. It keeps him from speaking lightly, insultingly of the suffering creature. Too many *explanations* are even more revolting – even more than evil itself, if that is possible – by their own brand of lightheartedness in which experienced pain gets short shrift, to the benefit of some artful sophism. Staying close to the wounded flesh, infinitely respecting its testimony, forgetting it all the less because it is silent in the agony of a little child or the groaning of a lowly animal, never wandering from the track of this experience, only daring to call on it with words that will be understood by the one who is suffering or who has suffered – all this is not an easy agenda. The language of revolt sometimes finds more tolerable words – we must dare to say and to admit it – than the language of apology. And even if we were to venture beyond revolt, trying to find another reality beyond, it would only be after having deeply adopted its movement, communicated with its spirit. Religious faith must be filled with an immensely delicate tact, a severe questioning of its own basis for action, before it can bear the wounded and revolted look of a man *who has suffered evil.*

Still a Reality for Man

Now I am emphasizing the thing in its raw nakedness. When I began, I clearly pointed out that evil is from the start something other than raw reality, that it includes history, civilization, man's self-assuming and secular attitude – *both* the question *and* the answer. Are my two assumptions not in irreconcilable contradiction? The truth is that evil, like pain, exists by reference to a raw, naked evil, comparable to the guarantee in back of paper money. But we will never know what that evil is; we are forever separated from it by our own selves. As the idea of "size," according to Socrates, enables us to distinguish something large from something small, so the matter of evil is the idea which serves us as a point of reference. The term "evil" is the *sign* at our disposition of that idea. We are not living on the immediate plane of naked reality, but on the mediate plane of symbols, communication by signs, obstacles. *And evil is signified on this very plane of things.*

Can suffering, as we have already asked, be distinguished from the knowledge of suffering? Is such a thing possible anywhere but at the very theoretical limit where consciousness pretends to be absent from the phenomenon, from which nothing can really ever keep it from being present? There is no more raw evil in the suffering of a small child than in that of a civilized adult. In a child we find an indivisible blend which should be given the composite name of "child's suffering plus participation of adult consciousness." The total participation of an adult, rebel or believer, is an *integral and undeniable part* of the child's suffering.

Whatever our desire may be to consider things objectively, "coldly," we are a part of the total situation, inevitably judge, prosecutor, and defendant. Such a remark is simple common sense but, nevertheless, it casts doubt on the objectivity, the reality, of an evil which is there before us and which would normally make itself felt, would cause suffering and would be qualified as an evil.

Before the arrival of man, conscious man, man and his *logos,* the world may have hypothetically resounded with cries and groanings, but they were *neutral. Before receiving a name, there is no evil.* Had it not been born, it would ever abort with the instantaneousness of a dream because there would be no consciousness, no time, no memory, and no word. The appearance of language produces communication by idea-bearing words which correspond to mixed realities, built up by man and time, diverse, all bearing the name of evil and by their diversity raising the "problem of evil." We are not always wrong in suggesting that our problems may be reduced to misunderstandings in vocabulary. But we would be in the wrong if we forgot that words contain different meanings because they carry in themselves the meaning of our experience, the totality of what we have become, shallow or profound, sceptics or believers.

Evil is born, then, for a being who can back off and look at his being as something apart from himself, and thus he judges as an observer. And evil is henceforth inseparable from both the judgment (implicit or not) *and* the thing judged. Thus man, with one act, both unveils *and* creates what life left in the folds of a total lack of differentiation. It has rightly been said that death exists only for man. Man is the being-for-death and in the same way the being-of-evil (in all the meanings of the term). Naming evil is creating it as an evil, that is, as a sign conveying meaning.

Evil is a reality for man and by man. Man is that being who can stop and back off, who can outline by the very direction of his look and by his attention select an image of the world, just as a child's eye suddenly catches the image hidden in the lines of a picture puzzle. The image is deformed not only by man's objectifying look, but also by his preference, partiality, and passion.

His look is centrifugal, transmitter rather than receiver, as we have already said with regard to perception and scientific facts.

Evil is a relation; it may only be understood in the unity of subject and object. It is impossible for me to reflect on an evil in which I am not implied as a mediator. It is impossible for evil to be an expression of the world without being an expression of man at the same time and vice versa.

From this unity of subject and object and the object's meaning for the subject, two main consequences may be derived which I will briefly enumerate here:

1. If experienced pain – suffering – cannot be separated from my reaction to it, it is therefore true that *somehow* an experienced evil must revert back to a committed evil (moral evil, sin). But this appears to be a scandalous assertion and merits some explanation. Let me say again that it is not sin, error, moral evil, or committed evil which has sparked this book; it is suffered pain, woe, the suffering of the world. Our only reason for speaking of the first category is because of its possible connection with the second. What could this connection possibly be? The two categories are often seen as two rivals throwing in each other's face the responsibility for events: is not suffered evil the consequence (the immediate sanction) of a committed evil? And is not committed evil the temptation of a victim who has fallen prey to the tempter and, therefore, a suffered evil? They can also be seen as the two faces of a single reality, of fundamental, original experience – suffered evil may not be isolated from my attitude nor, consequently, from my co-responsibility, from my reaction to that which I am suffering.

From this second viewpoint an objective evil has no meaning. There is no suffering passivity that is not blended in with activity, with a participation on my part, with a responsibility that is mine in this affair. However objective and bold we may pretend to be, we are compromised in the reality which we named in order to exercise it better, in order to meet it directly. We are mixed in with it. Evil *also* defines our partiality, our passion in the world. Or, from another angle, evil is an operative (or operational) concept. Only because man is not indifferent – not without differentiation – does evil exist. Evil defines the fact that we are different and tells how we are different. It defines our individuality and our revolt.

Does not the lack of distinction between suffered evil and committed evil, suffering and sin, originate in an archaic mentality to which it would only be to our disadvantage to regress since its only function seems to be to awaken old guilts buried in primitive man? I wish to make it known that my participation in what I call *evil* does not mean that I am guilty of my woes, that they are sanctioning my errors. In the two cases, "I have a part," but the differences between the meanings of the two cases must be carefully detailed.[9]

To make myself clearer I will take the concrete example of sickness. Disease is an evil, and no one can escape this obvious fact which would bring a smile were it not so weighty. The "powers of diminution," pain and functional helplessness, the whole cumbersome arsenal of disease, the waiting room of death – does not all this constitute an evil objectivity? However, pain is ambiguous. I have written elsewhere[10] concerning the ambiguity of illness, which resides in its double role as an *encounter* (it attacks me) and as a *sign* (on my ground and in my personal problems). And so it ceases being an external disorder, coming to me from the outside; it involves all that I am. Even more important it reestablishes,

[9] The disadvantages of the precritical confusion between pain and sin, and the decisive progress furnished by critical thought bring to mind certain remarks made by P. Ricoeur in the course of a meeting. It seems nonetheless that an ethical vision of the world is implied in the notion of evil and suffering, that evil is tied in with our liberty, even if man is not responsible for the origin of evil: "Even if evil were contemporaneous with the radical origin of things, it would nevertheless be true that only the matter through which it affects human existence makes it manifest." See P. Ricoeur, *Finitude et culpabilité* (Paris: Aubier-Montaigne), vol. 1, p. 14 [English translation is *Fallible Man* (Chicago: Henry Regnery Co., 1968)]. Is this not a way of tying together responsibility and situation? Cf. also Et. Borne: "Those distinctions, which from the beginning we suspect to be vain, between physical evil and pain, moral evil and error, metaphysical evil and the finiteness of what exists. . . ." Et. Borne, *Le problèm du mal* (Paris: Presses Universitaires de France, 1958), p. 30.

[10] Jacques Sarano, *Essai sur la signification du corps* [*The Meaning of the Body*].

in its own way, my broken equilibrium.[11] Illness is not only the expression of a disorder; it reestablishes order; it is a compromise, a solution, often onerous and the fruit of desperation, in view of healing.[12] Illness is an evil *and* a death-struggle against this evil.

This ambiguity prevents us from speaking of an objective evil, even that experienced in suffering. But this is no excuse for confounding, for no longer differentiating an evil to the point where we can no longer look it in the eye.

We must have the faculty of bringing evil before us – and of knowing that it all is not completely true. The precritical attitude magically confounds sickness, disorder, sin, and then multiplies evil by the sick guilt which it incites. The critical attitude shakes off this curse, exorcises this evil spell, awakes to the objectivity of evil as an adversary to be vanquished in hand-to-hand combat. This moment of critical opposition (technical, scientific, characteristic of our western civilization) is indispensable, and no one can intelligently bypass this moment of objectivity. When man is on his own feet, he has the right and the duty of setting evil and illness before himself as an object.

I have no right to attempt to go beyond this critical, objectifying phase until I have made room for it to stand up to an objectivity called evil. Then only may I ask myself how I could allow myself to be implied, compromised, to become a receiver, a co-participant in this strange, ambiguous blend of a reality. Just as illness is a blend of battlefield and aggressor (not everyone suffers from every germ), just as it is both sign and meeting-place, both an attitude of defense and of breakdown, so the evil of the universe is both what happens to me and the meaning I give it.

Evil is, on the one hand, what attacks me and what I try with all my strength to repulse. On the other hand, it is identified with this repulsion, this revolt which makes of it an evil and by this very opposition gives it its meaning in the universe. It is not a pure reality, but a reality pregnant with man's preference. The name he gives to it, the pejorative meaning he attaches to the name, seals his opposition and the position he has taken.

[11] This brings us back to the old theme of pain as a life-giving signal. The idea of sickness as a repairer of an evil is not entirely false, but must be stated with more nuances. Fever, faulty antalgic positions of the skeleton, etc., may occasionally be harmful, and we would be wrong in entrusting ourselves to the "common sense" of life. There are many defense reactions whose self-destructive blunders would merit the Freudian appellation of "death instinct." Fever kills. So do the "alarm reactions" (Selye) of the organism.

[12] Cf. Jacques Sarano, *La Guérison* [Healing], chapter 1.

This is a post-critical blend for it has not bypassed the dualistic moment of facing up to evil as an object and an adversary. It has no pretension of going back to the original undifferentiated state; neither does it aspire, on the pattern of poorly interpreted Hegelian synthesis, to situate everything in its proper place. Our only goal is, if possible, to take this paradox into account: Illness works against the life process and at the same time is included in it; evil may, in a certain sense, be identified with my revolt (my repulsion, my suffering), and yet it may be said that I am in revolt against it — as though it were there before me.

The truth is that I am unable to revolt against an objective evil — a second step, unless I have taken the first step of outlining it as an objective reality by facing up to what has happened to me. The I/world duality is the first act of refusal which in turn generates the world against which I then, and only then, am able to revolt. I cannot dichotomically say, "I revolt against THIS," unless I have already separated myself from THIS, by a breaking away which enables me to confront the world and is already a movement of revolt. Auto-position and opposition belong to a common cause. So the first step in my revolt is my dualism, and the revolt itself, the second step, results from the auto-position and the reduplication of the first step.

2. Another result of the unity of the object and of the subject is that as soon as the notion of objective knowledge gives way to the more concrete notion of experience, we will be forced to consider the problem of the *unity of empirical knowledge and of eschatological knowledge, of the scientific attitude and the religious attitude, of observation and of demand, of knowledge and of hope — the unity of hope and experience.* Here I am only mentioning considerations which will be the object of the last part of this work.

And "knowledge" of that phenomenon called evil, which I called a total intervention of man, is the expression and the visible form either of my cooperation or of my refusal to cooperate in a community, a creation from which it is impossible for me to remove or withdraw myself. Any knowledge is militant, both in its origins and in its effects.

There is a certain spectator's attempt at objectivity which only covers over the real complicity with the evil which it only was pretending to "observe." What I claimed to be observing is, in fact, my own work — because I deliberately purposed only to observe, and nothing else.

Evil is therefore a relation, a mediation, both by its goals and its results. It includes: *(a)* the subject/object relationship in both its original meaning and the genesis of its concept and *(b)* my relationship with the world and with God in its final meaning (the second step). It is origin and result in communication, one explaining the other. Let us say that evil is a mediation both when I propound the notion of evil and when I take my position regarding that notion. *Speaking of "evil"* is already an implicit judgment by which I repeat the first step, reduplicate it, and confirm that evil is a mediator between myself and the world, between man, the world, and God.

"The Champion of Observation"

If we wanted to make an inventory of the different ways of dealing with the "problem" of evil, of "handling" it, as we might say of a problem psychologically difficult to treat, we would have to begin our effort with a prologue announcing that we have already come to the last act. The concept of evil is a result, the result of stopping the projector so as to both project and immobilize an image of the world before man's eyes. But this objectivity is a singular one, for from the beginning it shows itself the accomplice of the reality it would like to know. "Evil be to him who evil thinks," goes the proverb. And, as a quip, we might say the same thing about the human eye. I emphasized this point earlier, and it is clearly not a question of insinuating that the world's suffering may be reduced to what man's look produces, but it only acquires its *meaning,* borne out by the name "evil," thanks to man's look, his realization of his own role. But his look is guilty, if I may say so, of abstraction, of analysis, and even more serious, of a critical attitude (in the two senses of the term), and of rebellion. Certainly man has not created evil, but by unveiling it he denounces it, points his finger at it as though it were an individual — like someone lost in the crowd who is suddenly recognized, surrounded — a personality called evil. So within this word we find man and his universe indissolubly implicated together.

An *inventory,* therefore, of the different ways of "handling" evil as a meaningful sign must begin by identifying the two *mute* attitudes, which say nothing about evil, by making them, forcing them to speak. For evil can only belong to a world which speaks, which expresses itself, which explains its own being.

I have already mentioned the first attitude of muteness, naked pain, which inexhaustibly nourishes the experience of evil, which is the original fountain from which evil flows and derives its scandalous existence. *But this pain is not evil;* it may never be; it cannot be evil until evil has, as it were, received its investiture, its advent, through recognition and adoption of responsibility by human consciousness. Evil is not, and cannot be, an *immediate* entity; it does not exist as long as it is wrapped up in ineffableness (or in an antepredicative attitude). It only becomes itself when it has gone out from itself and become something other than itself in order to give itself a name.

I have also mentioned the second mute attitude, that of refusal to accept the notion of evil, to take it into consideration, or to give it a visa (permission to reside). It is an indirect ignorance of evil. It is full of secret words which we could repeat, make public. Is it resignation, retreat in the face of scandal, pride hiding difficulties overcome, love afraid to make itself known? Faith and conformist hypocrisy can both hide behind this indirect ignorance of evil which claims to be initial and refuses to accord any meaning to the notion of evil, but which will have to admit that it is final, a result, a response — a response like all the others.

Continuing our inventory of the attitudes contained in the concept of evil we now reach the *objective attitude.* Its method is to observe evil dispassionately as it is, describe it, look the problem in the eye. This viewpoint is of the "scientific" type, but it must be included as one viewpoint among others. Evil appears to it to be the sum of all that suffers or fails in the world, but with a demand for perfection as its criterion, the demand for the "good" and the "beautiful" as asserted in "reason." Evil is considered as a deficiency, a deprivation, simply an attribute or an ornament of "good," the negative side of our inexhaustible desire to go beyond, that thirst never satisfied, always disappointed because it will be satisfied only at the end. When one set of requirements are met, this desire calls for more, and with that call is born the painful vexation which is called evil.

They call it the sum of all that suffers in the world. But does not this observation necessarily comprise a condemnation? How could one "objectively" sign the existence certificate of evil without at the same time recording its bad character? Here again the champion of observation has caught himself in his own nets. Evil will not permit such a separation. Unfortunately for objective analysis, evil is a *synthesis,* better suited for broad consciences than for narrow.

Observation in this case is condemnation. It provides the only definition of the word "evil": a synthesis of observation and condemnation, condemnation of creation, and hence of its supposed Author. It is *the identification of evil with human revolt.*

However, I must admit that the *"moment of observation"* does have its proper place. Observing evil, discussing its causes, presenting or refuting explanations for evil, putting God on trial or justifying him, perhaps concluding that a God of love and perfection does not exist — such are the thankless tasks of observation.[13] Defending the rights of objectivity, denouncing contradictions, tautologies, sophisms, *petitio principii,* hypocrisy hiding behind the usual explanations and justifications of evil — such is the task of the "champion of observation," in Kierkegaardian terms.

The analytical moment of observation endeavors to make a clear distinction between observation and assignment of meaning. It will perhaps accept, but only as a second step clearly distinct from the first, to find, to assign, and to transfuse a meaning into evil by the means of a demand which has clearly declared itself. This is only the second part, when the first has recorded that the scandal is scandal and the unjustifiable is unjustifiable. Observation and interpretation, then, are two different moments each of which refuses to be identified with the other, to be camouflaged by the other. The demand for interpretation, particularly, refuses to be confused with observation. I worked long at putting questions in their proper order, ousting unacknowledged desires for interpretation from their shelter of "innocent" observations. May observation speak its language and interpretation its own, but let there be no confusion between the two. Or if there is, we should at least be warned.[14]

[13] In concrete reality, all the "explanations of evil" are vain. But, as we shall see, it may be that their mistake is only in taking the form of explanations, whereas they bear witness to an inner requirement of man on an entirely different plane. The same misunderstanding paralyzes the discussion of "free will." The more these proofs collide with reality, the more they show up a valid experience which they are expressing but awkwardly betraying by the false language of "observation."

[14] One whole period of my life *(La modestie de Dieu* [God's modesty], *Le mythe de l'appauvrissement* [The myth of impoverishment] may be called my "moment of observation," that of my declarations against occultism. To better situate this period, here is a text written on August 29, 1949: "Only our acceptance and our love are fitting in the face of evil. But this is not because I have recognized in it any meaning or any worth. Any attitude which would suppose that there is in evil a hidden, incomprehensible, mysterious good is either shameful hypocrisy or unconscious gullibility. We must look evil squarely in the eye, not be ashamed of it, nor ashamed of God. For suggesting that God could not have wanted evil (either that he only wanted it for our good, or that he only wanted it through us) is being ashamed of God and lying to oneself instead of proudly assuming reality *as it is. We must admit the presence of evil.* It is legitimate to repulse it, to combat it, to hate it, to ignore it. But it is better

Let the veil of prejudice be cast aside to reveal evil face to face; for moral or religious demands for meaning camouflage, soften the scandal, conceal the difficulties. We must work, not from the postulates of faith, but from what *is*.

But we have already realized that the prejudice of pure observation is just as suspect in its demands as are the prejudices of religion or morality. It is illusory to try to separate observation from a decision against such an assignment by an espousal of a rationalistic prejudice. There is no impartiality. I used to think that faith betrayed the exactitude of the scandal of evil. But the absence of faith betrays it in the same way; they are just two forms of betrayal.

A determination to attain impartiality is hidden partiality. Separating a desire for meaning from observation is giving what will be called "observation" an abstract, biased form. This is so much so that it is perhaps more of a mistake to study evil without feeling a need (especially religious) for truth than with feeling such a need, for the simple reason that the desire to separate observation from this need is perhaps only a way of expressing my *absence* of faith.[15]

---

yet to hold out our hand to it, to go out to meet it, and to embrace it. This attitude asks more of us and in no way means that evil is somehow good. This attitude is superior to any other in the sphere of liberty. Liberty, if it can go high enough, reaches absolute disinterestedness, and beyond, love. So it will *finally* come out that the world is good after all. For our pride will allow us to assert it and believe it. We owe it to ourselves to assert it and believe it. If our pride can go through to the end, if our demands for truth reach the limit of love, we will then end up believing and asserting that creation is good in itself and not by our pride or our demands. Thus, *by an all-important detour,* we will come back around to the allegation which we at first called gullibility—that evil must really be a good and creation, despite the facts, is good. For, in effect, when our demands have passed over evil like a breath of air, the evil no longer exists: and this is truly so. It will, therefore, be true that there is no evil, that there must be none, *because* I must understand it, accept it, neutralize it by my very acceptance, as a base neutralizes acid. And this will be all the truer because my acceptance will be ignorant of its own work; *it will end up giving out as objective judgment the fruit of my infinite goodwill, of my stubborn, untiring prejudice in favor of love.*" Here is a living example of the turn which leads from an unindulgent objective observation to an observation/explanation, still dualistic, if I may call it such, and still emphasizing effort.

[15] In a mystery such as evil, there are so many unexpected ways of showing up one's faith or one's unbelief—from the most conforming assurance to confusion or revolt—that it would be unwise to claim the power of discerning the ground of faith from unbelief. Certain beatific optimisms are only refusals to think, screens thrown up to keep out reality. Some forms of calmness are only resignation; others are suppressed revolts. On the other hand, there are open revolts, disquieting and anguished states which are only openings, appeals.

So we must return to the critique of my method of knowing and speaking of evil. We would certainly be wrong in repudiating the good intention of trying objectively to state what is going on, of avoiding the collusion of occult demands. But if this objectivity consists only in "treating the world as an object," it loses its objectivity by its method of treatment (straight out of a chemistry laboratory). Its treatment has intervened just where it was forbidden to intervene. There is an objective knowledge which freezes the world and immobilizes "evil" in its evil form. This immobility of the world and "objectification" of evil are then only an expression of my attitude, of my refusal to advance, of my own isolation, and of my uncooperative prejudice.

Observation-knowledge is dead-weight-knowledge, a kind of pouting or boycotting of the world. It is like the ill will of someone who crosses his arms and looks on, who criticizes from his throne of nonparticipation. This observation is obstruction, opposition (in the sense of "offering opposition to . . ."), an act of sabotage against creation. Observation is a way of saying *refusal*.[16]

After, and dependent on, the spectator's knowledge comes cooperative knowledge, which gives of its own self. It is reputed to be a terrible enemy of evil. It destroys evil. Its intervention also concerns — no more, no differently from the preceding — the "object" of my knowledge and alters it. The very nature of this "object" evil is that it is necessarily transformed by the way I learn to know it and by the mutual action of the subject and the object.

In a more general sense, and even for the exact sciences since the appearance of the theory of relativity, *any knowledge is intervention.* The critique of that scientific knowledge claimed by the champion of observation has shown that my particular knowledge of a given item is a substantial part of its reality. The way I get to know it is therefore of the highest importance since it is an integral part of the reality which it desires to know. This is the age of the anti-dualism (or post-dualism, as you prefer) of knowledge, of unity in knowledge of subject and object. Such is the contrary of a dualistic conception which would juxtapose (like the gingham dog and the calico cat) subject and object in the act of

[16] Difficulty will come up again because of this refusal. It will be said that evil always reappears "somewhere," even if it is only in my decision to mention it or not to mention it! But as we shall see, the problem has changed; it implicates me; it *compromises* me to the evil that I wanted to objectify. And then the "committed evil" is incorporated into "suffered evil," whereas before the intention was to ascribe it to this second category. The dialectic of pain and suffering is renewed.

knowing and would reduce the object to a falsely abstract entity. This approach is not "relativism" or "subjectivism," but the perception of a *new objectivity,* no longer *a priori* or initial, but *a posteriori* and final, a result.

When on August 28, 1960, I took up again this critique which I had first written out on October 17, 1956, it seemed to me necessary to outline a "theory of partiality" as the condition for objectivity.[17] I roughed out the three following points: (1) We must be partial in order to render a healthy judgment of evil ("healthy" means "with all wisdom and with all truth"). (2) Our knowledge (of evil) is, in any case and in any hypothesis, partial, even when impartiality is claimed and desired. (3) But any partiality must in turn be "psychoanalyzed" and by the elucidation of all its details raised to the level of a new form of objectivity, of impartiality.

We must be partial before we can impartially judge evil. The first point presupposes that the second has been reached since it is first of all an avowal that the term, the experience, the notion of evil contains our partiality, our *passion,* and that an impartial view must include even that partiality. The word "evil" expresses, means, is one way of saying that *we are all in the same boat.* This is part of its very reality, we might say of its very essence. If we were not "all in the same boat," there would be no evil. It would even be contradictory and absurd to conceive of such a thing. The word "evil" implies from the first, by the very fact that we are using it, only observing it, that we are partial. The word "evil" means that we are both judge and defendant. The result is that *observing evil means* very clearly that *we are not observing,* but doing something more and something else.

True impartiality is conscious partiality, accepted and explicitly stated to be such.

Here is the other side of the coin: Partiality (in the negative sense of the term this time) is an attitude which claims to be, and believes itself to be, impartial—whereas it really is not, cannot be, will never be. He who claims to be the most impartial is the least of all. "Don't mix your fields," we are told. "Speak of one problem at a time; medicine, economics, religion, and then objectively, with the *appropriate method.* What are postulates about God or the meaning of creation and redemption doing here in a

[17] This "theory" of partiality will probably never come out, but nonetheless it has constantly reappeared in my writings (cf. *La culpabilité* [Guilt], *Médecine et médecins* [Medicine and physicians], and *Essai sur la signification du corps* [Meaning of the body]). (English edition of the latter is *The Meaning of the Body,* Philadelphia: The Westminster Press, 1966).

treatment of measles or stomach ulcers! Good working methods and scientific rigorousness require us to leave those things *out of the question,* to put them in temporary *limbo. . . ."*

"Leaving out of the question . . ." is a handy fiction which conceals two vices: *(a)* It is not what it claims to be; it disregards the postulate which is for all that no less present, but *which is not mentioned in the terms of the problem. (b)* This disregard throws out of kilter the very thing in question; if all the data are not mentioned, the problem is false. What does it matter then that such and such a solution is found? It will be fictitious, an idle tale with no account for life.[18]

Any judgment has its coordinates, its references either personal or historical. These may be considered either negatively or positively.

1. Negatively? Any espousal makes us less pure, and hidden motivations will be suspected for it, either from a psychoanalytic or from a Marxist point of view, as the result of a childhood problem or class conflict. It is no longer the support of a cause, a judgment, true or false, evaluated according to the criterion of truth. It is a symptom.

2. Positively? Here also Marxism shows the heuristic unity of means and of goals. Praxis concerns the whole man in the least of his so-called objective analyses. Dialectic has proved the falseness, for example, in economics, of the aphorism, "Science observes, does not judge." [19] A decisive criticism of the analytical spirit which "disregards" shows that I must partially (with a personal bias) reject this partial (incomplete) method because it is just as partial (biased) as mine but with the partiality multiplied by itself of ignoring or not being aware of its own partiality.

Criticism, therefore, will show that any observation which believes itself pure of partiality is the product of class or childhood conflicts — a sterile criticism, but not without its advantages. But if criticism went no further it would emasculate the possibility of any true judgment. It must advance its analysis another step and reach another objectivity more complete, by touching on and elucidating the elements *implied* in a judgment termed objective.

The objectivity which results is post-subjective, if I may com-

[18] Most of the criticisms of Teilhard de Chardin's work are inspired either by theological, philosophical, or scientific abstraction, which takes on the name of "rigorous method."

[19] Cf., for example: A. Pietre, *Economie et finalité* [Economy and finality], Cahiers de l'Institut de science économique appliquée, no. 99, (March, 1960), series M, no. 7.

pose the term. This new objectivity is no longer as superficially thin as it was in the type of judgment which "leaves out of the question . . ." in order professedly to order the questions better and get to the core of the problem. It is no longer that pseudo-scientific objectivity which is only a first approximation, emptiness, appearance, shadow, abstraction, or unreality. The new objectivity, not reached by the elimination of bothersome factors, but by their assimilation, offers henceforth the three-dimensional thickness of reality. It is experimental because it takes into account all of experience.[20]

So there are two ways of being partial, and there is no way of being impartial. One partiality consists in realizing one's partiality, the other in being unaware of it. Knowledge is reaching a neo-impartiality which is forever beyond the reach of the ignorance of partiality. The result, if such a thing is possible: Impartiality belongs to those who call themselves partial, and partiality is on the side of those who call themselves impartial.

Moreover, according to the opinion of the purest adherents of the analytical method, "leaving out of the question . . ." would dispense the observers from none of the factors implied in the process called "observation." On the contrary, the best analytical method would demand that every factor be examined. One who wants to eliminate "parasitical" factors (the personal coefficient) must operate by the same methods of inquiry before rejecting them as another does before accepting them. Both will agree on the capital importance of lucidly realizing and accepting what observation *implies*. Such an elucidation of our presuppositions, our partialities in the strictest sense would be inexhaustible. Objectivity is at the end – not initial, but terminal, not in the prologue, as with Descartes' rules, but at the end as in a conquest always

[20] May I repeat that it is Marxist analysis which renewed this meaning of totality, forgotten in bourgeois analysis, especially in economics. Against what is pejoratively termed "French Cartesianism," our day is insisting on the "thickness" of life as a part of objectivity, its phenomenological and existential depth. The individual, social, and historical factors are not eliminated but reintroduced into the problem and into the analysis itself. The objective attitude is a false objectivity. Its goal is to immediately eliminate all partiality, all passion, and all belief. But whenever a scientist has tried to stick to this challenge of "neutrality," he has passed judgments based on a conception of finality which he admitted to no one, least of all to himself. And his judgments were wrapped up in the very way he asked his questions, in the "Beware!" of his own neutrality. Thus every insistence on secularity is its own brand of clericalism. There is nothing more partial, more passionate than "neutrality." And some push this passion to a frenzy. And so science sometimes loses itself in extremes. The intolerant are killed by a profession of tolerance.

going on and never ended. Humility means never counting the last of my partialities, never finishing the avowal and the self-criticism of my presuppositions.

And my avowal itself is ambiguous: both an error and a victory, an inferiority and a superiority. And when (after naming it) I assert that evil is this or that, my words will be those of an unbeliever or a believer, my assertions will follow my class, my childhood filled with love or frustration. And everything which might have caused suspicion and perfidious denunciation has now become progress. Implication becomes the earnestness of advancement, and a disadvantage is transformed into fruitfulness.

An inventory of the ways of dealing with the problem of evil – themselves constituent elements of the reality in question – would furnish such combinations of evil and the person viewing the evil as: "evil-a-reality-for-the-man-in-revolt," "evil-a-reality-for-the-believer," for the rationalistic scientist, for the sentimental soul, or for the failure in life. Among all these it would be vain to try to isolate an "evil" (?) from the person who knows it. Knowledge is intervention. Observation is the expression of a desire for meaning. Evil is *more* than itself; it is the reality *of, by,* and *for* someone, an individual, an era, a world, a humanity. The essence of evil is that existence without an essence: evil-as-evil does not exist. Properly speaking, such is the case of any concrete reality. It involves, implicates, and compromises man's presence, his viewpoint, his life, and his responsibility.

It is impossible for me to think that pain (evil) exists and that I can really back off and look at it. My reduplication of self is a fake. My discursive reason acts out fictitiously what I cannot truly realize in the fullness of experience. The same is true of all the problems which are said to "affect us most closely." [21] If I take a position outside myself in order to objectify an evil in the world, this very duplication of self is a break, a segregation, an offense, and evil is the result of my fault. Duplicating self is constituting evil. We have called the unveiling of evil an ambiguity – for it is one element making up evil. My act of segregating myself from the world (from evil) makes me an accomplice of evil. Solidarity with evil is the result of that very act which helped to engender it, and this engendering of evil is due *both* to the intellectual act and the moral act. When separating myself from the world and evil, I cannot at the same time separate myself from the very evil which is

[21] Cf., for example, sexuality—I emphasize this aspect in my article in *Esprit* (November, 1960), especially p. 1852.

attached to my policy of separation. And I am implicated in the situation which I created by my separatist "observation," itself a position adopted with regard to life, a political act.

This is an inevitable, a necessary break even when I am denouncing it. Thus we are double, but never really double. I am so hard on this intellectual duplication of self only because its dwelling-place is in me. It is ever on the lookout for a way to trap me. It took up several years of my life. It is impossible to go beyond that through which we have not yet passed. The dualistic moment defines our incarnation, but betrays it at the same time.

The break is inevitable, on the level of our minds, but we must know how to assign its relative situation. When I observe that observation is yet something else besides itself, I pass beyond it also in an attempt to get back to beginnings, to the very womb of the concrete experience, to the ore which yields evil *before,* or rather *after* any extracting operation, any screening — after getting back to the before.

This reestablishment is what is ordinarily called "assuming" evil, or, what is the same thing, intervening actively and positively in the world, cooperating in action and hope. We will touch on this in greater detail in the last chapter. But the reestablishment can be turned around. The "objective" observation of an evil may be identified with a special mode of knowledge, what we shall call narcissistic knowledge because it is proof of a flaw in relations between the subject and an outside object (in analytical terms). The object of my words, of my problems, varies with the words themselves. Evil is not a fact; it is an experience. Any experience is testimony. Evil is my experience *and* my judgment of that experience. My judgment is an expression of my style of living in the world: It is testimony. This is why I can now risk this formula: Evil *is* my noncooperation with the world (*"is"* sums up all I have said: objective judgment and the observation of evil as such with an uncooperative mode of knowing). And here reappears the dialectic between suffered evil and committed evil, suffering and sin.

Two Dialectics of Sin and Suffering

"Suffering entered the world through sin." This is an unacceptable statement unless the speaker believes by faith, and an all-purpose faith, that evil can be conjured away by invoking sin and liberty. For many years I revolted, and correctly so, against this spiritual casualness so prompt at putting the responsibility for the world's pain on the shoulders of man and his sins. (I have since learned that this casual theological attitude is less widespread than I had thought.) For sin, even when joined by liberty, is a part of the world's suffering, of the calamities suffered in the world. Concerning *this point,* I have hardly changed over the years.[22] But I also considered it improper to take into account any previous commitments, any faith, improper to reverse the terms, as long as it was done in the name of a belief or religious faith. My leitomotiv was this warning: Do not present as an observation the results of prior requirement (that of religion or of love, etc.).[23] The differentiation between sin and evil, which some pretend is so decisive in the history of the world, was never so harshly stated as at the critical age of my life.

Today — how things turn! — the insulting formula, "Pain came into the world by sin," bothers me less:

1. Because I have realized that personal attitudes (love, religion) may only awkwardly be explained by arguments and proofs, in terms of observation (as we will see in the next chapter);

2. Because, on the other hand, I am more wary today than I was then of observation. No longer can I conceive of observation which is not the expression of an attitude of love or non-love, whether or not it is admitted or even conscious. Hence, *suffered evil* is inseparable from a kind of complicity on my part, from a kind of committed evil in its vaguest and most inclusive sense.

Whence the two dialects of pain and sin.

The first juxtaposes them, and in a process carried out on a psychologically primary level, "objectifies" evil, imputes its responsibility to pain. Or, answering offense with offense, it imputes sin to suffered evil. This abstract method is based on notions of causality. You are suffering because you have sinned.

In fact, my participation in the pain of the world (and in my own) is more subtle than that. The second dialectic of suffering and sin does not play the game of massacre by mutual imputations: It admits that pain and sin are inseparable — and thus comes back to an unlettered lack of differentiation between evil and sin which some might call a regression. They are inseparable for the oft recognized reason that the very observation and declaration of evil as something bad requires more than my suffering; it requires the "account" (Goldstein), hostile or friendly, that I give of my relationship with the world.

[22] See the next chapter, devoted to the *explanations* of evil.
[23] See note 14 in this chapter.

This is why the experience of pain is not the same for the man in revolt and the wise man or the believer. For each it is a different experience in the deepest and most immediate depths of his body. For the body is inseparable from my overall attitude and from my style of existence. Evil is inseparable from its *meaning,* that is, from the way it is *utilized* (and so I take up the old moralities of pain), even when it is most catastrophically experienced in my flesh or in the suffering and death of a child. The experience of someone like E. Mounier was one with his child's pain; it was a whole which it would be entirely false to dissociate into two phases — observation, then the requirements of the individual. It is a totality, a single movement as simple as the gesture of a hand. Suffering/faith is just as real, just as legitimate, in any case, as the suffering/revolt of the unbeliever who also suffers cruelly from the same wound. It would be an insult, and incorrect, to insinuate that one's suffering is so easily turned back by faith only because the wound is felt less cruelly, unjust to speak of happy unconsciousness, of resignation, or even of indifference or hypocrisy.

Only the analytical attitude, a valid attitude, can separate observation from individual requirements. In concrete reality they are always present together. The alternative is not a choice between the two, but between the two combinations mentioned above. Why have I chosen "segregation-knowledge" rather than "cooperation-knowledge"? On this choice depends the very *reality* of the evil I confront. It would be just as true to say that my attitude is motivated by evil and that evil is the result of my attitude.

Thus it is easy to understand how evil can be engendered by me in two ways:

a) by the evil things I do, moral evil as it is commonly viewed; or,

b) by what I put into the term "evil."

Such is the double dialectic of sin and pain.

The Ontology and Phenomenology of Evil

Evil is more than itself, because it is inseparable from me. In the idea "evil" I doubly express that I am interdependent with the world: The world and I are "in the same boat," either by cooperation or by noncooperation. And I contribute doubly to evil: by my evil actions, and by my vision of the world which in one way or another includes evil as a meaningful entity.

However, such an anti- or post-dualistic attitude has no more right than any other to assert itself dogmatically, and my criticism in the 1950's of the collusion between observation and personal attitudes, between psychology and ethics, is still valid.[24] As concerns the present study, this means, may I recall,[25] that whether we like it or not, evil does exist, really and cruelly, and it is not my way of looking at it or the weakness of my judgment which gives it reality. This also means that the unity of subject and object, of personal attitude and observation, does not eliminate another objectivity, which in its turn dualizes or decomposes my manner of living into observation and personal attitude.

For is it not necessary, in order to truly understand that I include myself in my most objective observation, that I be able to separate the inseparable and become conscious of my own duality? But this duality will *change positions* during the process. It was that of observation and the personal requirements of fact and worth. But it may become that of unbelief and faith, the one insisting on confronting evil with no mitigating circumstances, no excuses, no context, the other considering it in the center of a totality including our Father and his Son.[26]

In this problem we are studying, we find, as elsewhere, two viewpoints, one concerning being, the other dealing with meanings.

Thus from the beginning, evil may be considered as a reality affecting the being. For example, it is what excludes being; it is deprivation of being. Evil is not a being; it is the lack of being. In religious terms, evil is what goes against the will of God; it presupposes a liberty capable of opposing divine omnipotence. In anthropological terms it is what hinders the realization of our calling in life (our "nature," our "finality"). In cosmological terms it is designated as obstacles to the realization of the world considered to be oriented toward a goal. Having thus endowed evil with an ontological status, the next step is to seek out its causes and its results. From this point of view, evil exists independently from man's conception of it, from human judgment, which is only the observation of a reality, reflection on a reality.

[24] Cf., for example, "La liberté chez Descartes" [Liberty in Descartes' writings] and "Le pouvoir de refus" [The power of refusal], in *Etudes philosophiques,* no. 2 (1950) and no. 3 (1952).

[25] See p. 107.

[26] This is how I looked on this dialectic of observation and personal requirements in 1954: "Any observation is certainly revealing of a personal attitude (of a person's deepest purpose), but the opposite is also true. Any personal requirement is necessarily an object to be observed. A fact is evidence of a preference, of an assignment of worth, and in turn, worth is a fact to be observed by the scientist. Respect for observation as such is a demand. As soon as subordination to personal attitudes is openly declared, these attitudes disappear in observation."

We have already faulted this point of view for disregarding human judgment just when it is asserting itself by using the name *evil.* All the preceding definitions are not analytical, but synthetical. They are composed judgments, dealing with an ideally immediate family, which no one, of course, would dream of contesting, which we have called raw pain, but which is not evil. Evil is here already endowed with a meaning. It is, moreover, a negative meaning, as we shall see, but one which, in any case, implies an irreversible humanization of the raw fact. Under these conditions, how is it possible to give evil ontological status without going through the necessary intermediary of a phenomenological treatment which would deal with meanings? Although we would be the last to contest the legitimacy of a metaphysics of evil, we, nonetheless, believe that it must make its way through the interworld of meanings before one day emerging, but still with difficulty.

A beginning must be made, however much that may cost in *experience,* in my personal experience of pain and of evil, which means, like it or not, that this experience will be a complex one: illness, the death of someone dear, or participation in the suffering of a friend or of a child. It will include both a fictitious "immediacy" and, inseparably, my position, my "negation," with respect to it. The negation itself includes a great number of interrelating details, conscious or unconscious. Every pain, including that of a small child, implies the participation of consciousness in order for it to acquire the significance of an evil. In a desert this child's groaning calls forth no echo, has no meaning: It is nothingness. We see it as an evil because, and to the extent that, we are *present* (even if we suppose we are absent).

Evil has no status distinct from the human consciousness that judges it, which condemns it. Evil cannot be distinct from human revolt. Speaking of evil is the same as speaking of condemnation and revolt. But the opposite is also true: Evil has no status distinct from reality, that is, from the *contents* of our revolt, of our condemnation.

It is only afterwards, by the process of a painful restoration, of a conversion, that we cease identifying evil with our condemnation of it. Only then can it be situated in a cosmological or theological totality. And it is then, and only then, that an ontology of evil may be elaborated as a synthesis of subjectivity and objectivity, of judgment and of being. For such an ontology may be obtained through a totalization of our experience. It becomes more objective and more concrete, and we believe that the result of this objectification, of this concrete totalization, will be to *situate* meaningful evil in being, expressed as a doctrine, I will even say, as a theology. It is only the result of a difficult and time-consuming effort. Accepting such a solution from the beginning as though it were self-evident would be passing over real difficulties, supposing them resolved by others, not taking the trouble of scaling the steeps that no one else can scale in our place.

I believe, therefore, that it is impossible to dispense with the slow and difficult progression which takes us from meaning to an ontological status. Only by a slow genesis and growth of consciousness can meaningful evil (judgment, condemnation, revolt) reach the end point of a reality which is a part of being. The process is one of maturation that might be overlooked in the logical order of exposition although it is the essential point, a journey accomplished as a personal experience and lasting till the voyager attains a total vision of creation as Creation.

It is true that evil is a judgment, and also true that it is reality: inseparably both. Evil is judgment passed on reality and a *judgment dealing with a reality. It is neither a reality without this judgment, nor a judgment without this reality.*

Considering evil to be a reality is an error, for the reality which we have just delineated is below the level of what is qualifiable and thus not yet evil. Considering evil as an opinion is also an error, but a partial one which bogs down on the critical level, at the dualistic level, at the level of dualism of appearance and essence, of the phenomenon and the noumenon. We must go beyond this stage. Progress, if you wish, from Kant to Hegel, and propose that evil is judgment passed on something that *is, and its reality includes the judgment I have passed on it.* This reality only comes to light because of my consideration of it, and hence my consideration is a part of its essence. After a Kantian dualism comes a Hegelian synthesis and a metaphysics which is not initial but terminal. The end result is the status of evil in being which, far from excluding it, includes the presence of the human subject. Evil is a mixture of subject and object. And we can now understand how it exists *by* us just as much as *for* us, and how it has, at the same time, or at least begins to have, its own existence. I express the evil that is, and I give evil its being. I contribute to it by my analytical, objectifying intervention, like a catalyzer speeding up electrolysis.

What appears, then, is a dualism within a monism. Evil is the expression of a fault in being, an internal division, "something" which permits the appearance of evil. Man himself is the most striking witness of this fracture within his being, because of his dualizing nature, itself a bearer of division. His language, his power, and his liberty are ways of expressing, in images and as clearly as broad daylight, his auto-opposition, carried out within his own being. I oppose my own being, and by so doing I am also a spokesman for my being, its messenger.

Evil is both an *expression* of my being and my opposition to this being. Any symptom or any sign is also expression and opposition to the extent that this expression, sprung up like a bud from reality, is distinguished from that reality and is henceforth counted as a part of reality – one of its fruits.

Because it is both emanation and opposition, evil is ambiguous. That is why, on the one hand, people can wander around blindly and say anything they want about it. But on the other hand, it is impossible to say entirely what one wants to say without raising protests and indignation from the human consciousness.

Judging is proclaiming what is. But it is also announcing something *about* what is. This is why there is a possible spread, a margin of error, between the judgment rendered and what *is*, a margin which is removed by truly human participation.

An ontology of evil, gained by phenomenology, must be rooted in a concrete progression, in a growing experience, which is the result of my suffering, of our universal suffering.

Evil and Human Revolt; a Critique of the Absurd World

Evil expresses a relation. It includes something else and something more than we would tend to see in the word itself. This is why the laborious work of setting out the explanations for evil, in order to assume or reject responsibility for it, must come after a period of ascetic analysis of what is implied in the idea of evil and in our compromising which it reveals.

Evil puts me in a situation of compromise because it is the subject giving meaning, the author of concepts and judgments. Evil is other than naked pain; it is also a condemnation which bears within itself its own seed.

I repeat here a sentence from my study *La culpabilité* [Guilt] (1957): "Evil is a category of human revolt, which in turn is a category of guilt."[27] A paradoxical reversal: of course, I rebel be-

[27] Jacques Sarano, *La culpabilité*, p. 17. The whole first chapter of this book is a reply to the particular aspect of the problem of evil which I am now presenting.

cause of evil, but that is seeing only the superficial succession of appearances. Evil appears in turn as the result of my revolt and accusations. The problem of evil is thereby included and transcended by the more comprehensive problem, the more general notion of guilt, which implies man's judgment and his demands for justification.

This is another way of stating the same truth: I am implicated in the problem of evil whether I am a believer or a nonbeliever, as a man in general, able to turn against what he is suffering, to move away from it and to get his wits about him – in order to judge and condemn, accuse and denounce. Speaking of a subject/world relationship is not enough; evil expresses a relationship on an ethical plane and, especially, on a religious plane. This relationship not only implies a subject, but a subject oriented by ethical and religious considerations. The word "evil" has meaning only for a subject and a subject for whom the world itself has meaning. For the world can only be without meaning for someone who would require of it a meaning, and in whose eyes the world must have meaning.

I will term the following lines a critique of the "absurd world." For if the world had no meaning, it would be impossible to state its lack of meaning. Speaking of evil is bearing witness to Absoluteness. Even better, being concerned about evil is bearing witness for a God of love.[28]

It is impossible to imagine clearly enough the nobility of a world

[28] This idea that God—even the Judeo-Christian personal God—is implicitly, and however much it may be denied, contained in our very protestations which deny or ignore his existence; this oft forgotten but nevertheless classical idea still appears to some as nothing but a scandalous sophism, a rape of the rebellious conscience, of absurd or atheistic man in whose mouth some would like to put words that go beyond what he is clearly and distinctly saying.

For the atheistic mind, it is just as false to allege that a world without God is neutral (neither good nor bad) as it is to assert that a world with God would necessarily be good.

But we must not sell off too cheaply the other levels or facets of human contestation:

1. Considered from the aspect of a mystical *doctrine of happiness* (elaborate or not), man would call it a "dog's life." The why or the against what are of little matter! The immediate feeling is enough, the abrasion of everyday life.

2. Considered from the viewpoint of an *ethics of justice* (elaborated or not), suffering for a victory would be valid, but not unjust suffering. What is the basis for the division? It is conscience, raised to the level of an absolute.

Even if God is implied by this absolute (as he is twice over implicit, if I may say so, in the exclamation, "It's a dog's life!" and in man's appetite for happiness), we must not neglect to emphasize that the *conscience* is still a necessary intermediate (even for the believer). Without this mediation of the conscience (the common ground where believers and nonbelievers can get to-for which evil exists as evil. As we have already said, suffering and destruction are neutral, with no quality, as long as they have not been qualified. But man stands up, takes all of that in hand, and judges it. He causes one thing to be *evil,* another *good.* And we may now understand all that the present condemnation of the world in the term and the idea of "evil" implies, its connotations

---

gether and communicate), there is a terrible risk of a religion without morals, totalitarianism, the religion of an authority or pure force called God.

We could not emphasize too much how important this remark is and how many snares each step of its *formulation* must avoid. When I say that God is *implied* by the protests of affectivity or conscience, I have no intention of burying in silence, of passing over the different levels (or stages) in each person's realization of these problems. Thus when I occasionally refer to Jesus Christ by name in this book, as I have done in others (cf. *The Meaning of the Body),* it must be very clear that I am not forcing someone who speaks another language than mine to accept this name as truth. What I am saying is that the basic truths persist, however one may live them, think them, or speak them. The work of growth which I call the work of Jesus Christ in each of us and in all of humanity is being accomplished just the same whether it is stated in those terms or others.

Some (rigid theologians) proclaim the law of all or nothing. The only thing that counts is an explicit faith in Jesus Christ. Any other religious, or *a fortiori* moral, quest is far from a stage, a preparation, a stepping-stone—it is nothing.

On the other hand, religious syncretism homogenizes all religious quests or doctrines and thus abusively relativizes the truth of revelation.

Between these two extremes, Christian tradition teaches that Christ is a universal power for salvation, that he is present and working, leavening explicitly each one of us. But he is in each person (and civilization) according to each person's own degree of growth, of explicit adhesion, and of realization of the divine manifestation. It is absolutely necessary to *respect* in each person the degree of motivation he has achieved, never to substitute oneself for another's conscience or his language.

The "holy heathen" worked in Christ without knowing him. The prophets believed (implicitly) in Christ who was only being announced, but the announcement took in the announcers. And the concept has been correctly stated as a "Christian sense of the Old Testament."

The notion of "providence" is a means of designating this implicit presence of Him in whom we believe in the midst of the heathen, and the work of purely moral virtues (the meaning and the demand for justice are understood by us as revealers of Christ's implicit presence).

But every individual names this demand, this presence, this growth according to his own conscience—which absolutely must not be forced. An apparently orthodox formula does not mean much; on the other hand, its explanation may be far behind the *life* of God in someone. Flaunting the *letter* of religious faith is scandalous under these circumstances, as though we wanted to play the judge, to "show off" our piety. There is no need of elevator service up to Jesus Christ. He must be met in the progress of maturation, each individual must retrace the steps of the history of salvation as found in the Bible.

Each of us, if we want to be in the truth, must respect in others (and demand that the same respect be given him) the *stages of truth* and the form truth will take in the consciences of different people.

of *humanity* and *beyond* (super-humanity, I mean, divinity, eschatology).

The idea of evil can be conceived only by the human mind. It reveals a mind capable of endowing something with the quality of bad or good. And by this human judgment it reveals a strange requirement, that of perfection.

This condemnation goes back to a *reality* from which the human mind draws insatiably, which nourishes it, without which it would be incapable, would have no means of judging some things evil — sufferings or destructions, not even the worst of them. The notion of evil is born only when a certain degree of civilization and of human maturity has been reached. This landmark of reality, by which evil may be designated and condemned, is the reality of goodness, without which nothing could be bad. That indication of goodness is proven by evil, as imperfection has been called an evidence of perfection. "What we in our experience call justice or love is only such because it verifies or expresses something about an aspiration toward, or the presence of, that virtue. . . ." [29]

Speaking of evil is providing evidence of *that reality* which situates, which transcends it, and which denies it. In this sense (as with scepticism), a condemnation asserts what it denies. In other words, it goes beyond that *reality* which it is condemning. Recognizing evil is both constituting it *and* denying it.

When we revolt, we are therefore giving proof of our need for the divine. Man must necessarily have kept something divine in him (a Platonic "reminiscence" of divinity) in order to be capable of revolting against certain events in this world — famines, earthquakes. Such kind of nostalgia is in itself a confession — a nostalgia without which evil could never have been defined or identified.

We cannot lend too much importance to the theme, just as scorned as overused, of *the optimism implied by the notion (and the condemnation) of evil.*

It is impossible not to take into account the kind of faith *implied or denied* by the man in despair, the unbeliever, the "absurd man" who, from Dostoevski to Camus, has never forgiven Creation for the horrible sight of a small child in pain. If the suffering of a child did not stand out against the assertion that there should be no such thing, if it did not stand out against a world it insults and which is therefore worth something, if it did not stand out color for color against a background entirely different from itself, such

[29] G. Madinier, *Conscience et signification* [Conscience and meaning] (Paris: Presses Universitaires de France), p. 89.

pain would not shock us, would not revolt us. It would only run up against our indifference; it would skirt our unconsciousness, our complete lack of consciousness to its abnormal and revolting nature. Pain only insults a world which *merits* being insulted. And if the world did not send me back to *someone* to whom I can speak, if it had no meaning for me, it would not even merit being condemned; a suffering child could not even make it ashamed.

So I repeat my initial proposition: *"If the world had no meaning, it would be impossible to state its lack of meaning."* The rebel who denies that the world has any meaning is an impenitent optimist, a "spiritualist" who does not know himself. This unbeliever is a believer more demanding, more serious than any of our sheep so easily satisfied. This unbeliever is more in love with God and more jealous of rivals than any of the "faithful" so rapidly satisfied with "explanations" for evil. God loves rebels. He loved Job, against the pious solicitude of his friends.

The second corollary of the same proposition: A world without God could not be "bad." Denying God because of evil is asserting with those very words that he is present and active; it is only denying him with a rejection, after having admitted his existence. Negation of God, if it were logical, would saw off the branch on which it is sitting.

It would be proper, then, to come to an agreement about the kind of "atheism" to which revolt against universal pain would lead. This atheism makes the presence of God absolutely necessary; it summons him to the defendant's bench and obliges him to explain his actions. Evil means not only that something has happened but that I condemn that thing and pass judgment on God. Evil is man judging God – even when his judgment is turned as a punishing sword against him (our suffering because of our sin). And it is not God's inexistence which frightens us, but his silence, which is even more terrible. And his silence supposes that he is there, alive, present and absent, like a debater who is vainly trying to elude the question and whose last leg must be cut from under him. This God is particularly close, singularly human and personal, and in a certain (incomplete) way singularly Judeo-Christian. The Psalms are cries for help and cries of revolt. A God purely transcendental would not have engaged in the combat of Jacob with the angel, confrontation and trial that it was. We must admit that the God called to trial by the man rehabilitated by Camus under the name of man in revolt or *absurd man* – there is no other valid image of man in revolt – singularly resembles the Judeo-Christian God who is supposed to love us, hear us, and speak to us, but does not speak to us, who is supposed to take care of us, but abandons us. And we carry on bitter discussions with him, as did Moses and the prophets. The God whom we are bringing to trial because of evil can only be the God of the Bible and of the covenant, who swore an *oath* with regard to creation and its creatures, as we have bound ourselves with regard to him. A singular atheism!

Evil means accusing God.[30] Accusing God, if I dare say it, is doing him the honor of believing in him, of considering him as a (valid) Person to converse with, someone near to us, accessible to dialogue, to justice, to an exchange, and to love.

So we can cry out to the absurdity of the world, "You have to be two" (as we so easily say in joking, "You have to be two to get married").

Evil does not cast doubt on God's existence but on his *nature:* Who is such a God, both Creator and Father, who *permits* (only permits, unless we should say desires) such things to happen? Without God there can be no evil. Evil is my confrontation with God, which means that I have approached God. The figure of Job is the most pathetic answer to the figure of God that exists.

The idea of evil implies with the same imperative proof both the double presence of God and man and their disagreement as concerns the world. Evil is the relationship between God and man, his creation.

Evil is an argument between God and his creation concerning the world. Evil is the name which we have given to their grave dissent with regard to the world.

Although the issue is between God and man, unfortunately the conversation is almost always a monologue by man. The rare occasions in which God intervened are to be found in the Bible. Doubtlessly God also reveals himself indirectly, by an event, an act, or a sign whose meaning we were to grasp: Christ's coming. Of course, this sign is meaningful only for those who know how to read its account and who accept its context. But were we not already implicitly in this context when we chose the word "evil," its meaning, and its agonizing mystery? This we have emphasized enough. But it was proper to remind ourselves of it. Since evil as a sign only exists in a context of personal religion, lest it be reduced to an inconsequential entity, we must not abandon its prem-

[30] It is now easier to understand my apparently paradoxical phrase in *La culpabilité*, p. 17, quoted earlier: "Evil is a category of human revolt, which in turn is a category of guilt."

ises; we must follow their logic to the end. And if we have, perhaps in spite of ourselves, begun a dialogue with God, we must listen for the signs which he might possibly send us. Answering that these signs have no value for "unprepared" minds is forgetting that man and neutrality are mutually exclusive, for man is the being that destroys the world's neutrality (virginity). Without man's intervention the world cannot attain evil (good and evil). Neither is it possible without a personal God, good and perfect. There is no evil unless we have beforehand attributed this world to a God *from whom we were expecting something else.* What goes beforehand is extremely important. There is no evil as such, unjustifiable, unless we first believe in God, and unless we have a precise picture of what God is. He is disappointing because we first saw him with specific features. And unjustifiable evil is only possible because of a demand for justice presupposed in man and expected of God.

The trial of God (that is, the idea of evil) is pessimism grafted onto a deep-rooted optimism. It is despair nourished on a disappointed hope, a hope asking only to be reborn, despair between two hopes. This could give the deceptive appearance of a hasty end to our quest. How?

Evil is the place where God and man meet in confrontation. This confrontation is only conceivable and realizable if it is the result of a real presence, and a double presence, of God in man and man in God: a double love which has been disappointed, a concrete disappointment. Two "whys" come from man's lips, in two phases. They will furnish the subjects of the next chapter and the last chapters of this book.

1. The first "why" could be called the *why of origins,* because it is always prodding and digging into evil in quest of its possible origins. Man wants to force God into an explanation of the causes of evil. This is the judgment phase, the explanation phase, the phase of causality, of rationalism, of revolt, which is nothing other than the phase of observation I mentioned earlier, the moment of separation, of dualistic and critical objectification. This spirit inspires the more or less ingenious "explanations" of evil, with a kind of "clearing God of guilt" in mind. It also inspires a legitimate disdain for such explanations when they are read in the spirit of causality. We shall see all this in chapter 2.

2. The second "why," the *why of ends* corresponds, if you wish, to the phase of reconciliation. All explanations seem ridiculous, for this is the moment of comprehension. This comprehension is not concerned with the "why" of evil's origins or its initial cause

(although it does sometimes blunder into the language of causality, as we shall see, but it would be best to understand this symbolically, a story told to illustrate a hidden truth), but with the final "why," not with *knowing* but with *doing* (cooperating). Speech will express in its own way a reciprocal *act* of love from man toward God, in response to and patterned after God's act of love toward man. Hope and redemption are the categories of this phase of the conflict which we will try to present, to the extent that such a thing is subject to explanation, in the last chapter.

Before being capable of a serene judgment of evil, as we have said, man must be partial and passionate. And I would add that he must be partial; he must necessarily side with God. Jeremiah expressed this passionate partiality:

> "Righteous art thou, O Lord . . .
> Why does the way of the wicked prosper?"

Whatever the consequences may be, even though they lead to logical contradiction, God is righteous. We can deal with the difficulties afterwards. For now, I'll take God's side. I am conscious of what I am doing and in good faith I assert that I am partial *with* God. I must admit it and assert my partiality as it is. Putting forward "logical arguments" [31] is another way (but unconscious or hidden) of manifesting the same passionate attachment, of concealing the fact that unshakable postulates have already been adopted, and of unveiling at the end of the discussion what had already been accepted before starting: the righteous God, whose resemblance to the Judeo-Christian God I have already mentioned. The argument game is purely on the surface while the adversaries are really on the same side, whether they know it or not. The problem of evil is a "one-party" problem (like some elections). We do not have the possibility of making an unprejudiced choice between two parties. Before I even begin, I am working on the hypothesis of a just God, from that moment and because of the very fact that I am accusing him of injustice. I would not accuse him of such a thing if I were not counting on his being just, and so paradoxically I deprive myself of one of the most "logical" conclusions of evil — that we are subject to a God of injustice. Such is the paradox of evil: It makes us assert what we deny and makes us worship the One against whom our vehement pain cries out its revolt.

[31] As we shall see in chapter 2 of Part II, the "explanations" of evil use the poor judgment of proposing arguments as "logical" as, "If God is all-powerful and complete goodness, why does he not put a stop to pain?" (as an answer to "If God were infinite and perfect, he would not have wanted evil to exist").

The moments of explanation and of comprehension are inseparable. This anticipating remark was only put here to show to what extent it is important for me to understand that no one can pose the "problem of evil," and even less solve it, unless he presupposes the existence and presence of God. Although God is guilty of being absent, he is nevertheless just and good, even if he is incomprehensibly lacking in goodness. Concluding from evil that God does not exist is senseless. It would be better to say, "The God I had represented in my own mind does not exist." [32] It is my image of God – all too human – which is in doubt. That changes everything. If *speaking of evil is a way of speaking of God* (like it or not), we must also add that it is inseparably a way of speaking of man: "Who is God for me? What terms am I on with him? What is my relationship with him?"

I shall have to define a whole *diplomacy* in my relationship with God, in my life, and, more particularly, in the experience of pain for others and for myself. Here then we come back to the two attitudes which we said had to precede the constitution of the "problem of evil." We realize that evil may not be attacked directly, in itself and as itself. It implies a great number of hypotheses or attitudes which concern myself and God, our relationship, and my relationship with myself and with the world (the other aspect of my relationship with God).

Following my attitude of hostility or of confidence, whether I cut myself off from the world or accept my solidarity with it and give God the benefit of the doubt, the "concept" of evil changes completely. Have I isolated myself like a stone stranded on the bank of a stagnant pond while the current flows on a few feet away? Am I dead (weight); am I in a state of passive resistance? Evil is the stone I cannot swallow. Rigid as it is, the philosophy of contradictory explanations of evil is a single-plane discussion – critical, objective, sterile – whose contradictions are fatal, whose discrepancies are insoluble. Two-dimensional space is an incorrect medium for representing the true relationships between total man and the world. It is the static space of "whys" all the way back to the causes and origins, of condemnations, of refusal to accept responsibilities.

But when I get into the action, when I play the game (let us compare it to the renewal of action in "The Night Visitors"), then

[32] P. Ganne calls him, "Our little portable God"—made more for our use than in our image.

this deadly contradiction ceases; the "problem of evil" loses its force and is solved by my action, accomplished in the pursuit of creative and laborious liberty. Work is a solution for the problem of evil. The problem is solved for the simple reason that it is stated in other terms. Earlier I said that stating it is implicitly solving it in one way. And here we have come to the same conclusion: "Evil" is a word that says how we understand or do not understand the world and, more exactly, God's creation. In a world without God, as in a discussion between men who do not know God, "evil" is a group of letters deprived of all meaning, empty.

To conclude, I would say that an inquiry into evil must be made with reference to an inquiry into the bases of that inquiry; such are the indispensable prolegomena to the problem of evil. Evil is not an immediate phenomenon; it implies the fact itself of evil and its meaning; and meaning means relationship.

1. "Evil" does not have to do only with this universe, but with the blend of human consciousness and the world, that world where man is present, capable of judging good and evil, that is, of judging creation and God himself. Man is a part of it all; he implicated himself when he spoke the word "evil."

2. Evil does not have to do only with the world but with the blend of the world as it is and as it should be. This is another relationship, but this time with the absolute as one extreme. An absolute which has a name, which is a person: The belief in this absolute, like it or not, consciously or not, is a belief in the Judeo-Christian personal God. Evil may be a proof that God does not exist — but the very fact of speaking of evil would be impossible if God did not exist!

Evil is a relational concept, and its meaning everywhere overflows the content of its own literal meaning. Pain in the world has no *intrinsically* negative quality. That quality originates elsewhere, and the *elsewhere* is of capital importance. It indicates exactly that which was not first expressed in the notion of evil and which we have tried to make clear: *(a)* that we transcend and *deny* evil by our very possibility of qualifying it, of situating it; by this very action we are *elsewhere,* we bear evidence of a spiritual reality which originates *elsewhere; (b)* that the world itself transcends and *denies* the evil to which it has given birth. That is, the world is directed as a vector is directed. Like a boat, its prow is pointed in one direction. That is what we call a *creation.*

Therefore, evil is both (1) a sign that we are spiritual beings; (2) a sign that we are created beings, participating in history, in the work of a Creator. Without him, evil is an empty word. It would be just as empty if the God in question were an abstract God, a metaphysical God, instead of our personal God, our Father.

We hear it said that evil is a scandal. It would be better to say that it is the expression of a scandal, a vexation, a disappointment, and therefore a confrontation of two orders: the linear world of empiricism, on the one hand, and the world of religious demands, on the other. *Evil is therefore the synthesis of a demand and an observation*. Observation alone is not enough. Evil is not observed, then stated. It is the connecting line between two experiences, between two planes. Without such dualism, it would have been impossible for pain to change over into the problem of evil.

When we get around to speaking of those processes which claim to *observe* evil and reflect on it in order to justify it and see in it a scandal or a mystery, I hope that the preliminary remarks developed in this chapter will furnish the climate indispensable for the understanding of the ideas developed there.

2

The Vanity of Explanation—Apology and Rebellion

The champion of observation, as we presented him in the last chapter, bravely argues about evil, examines the pros and the cons, and tries the strength of every explanation without trying to see beyond the goal, the demands of which the explanation itself is in its own way evidence.

So we greatly needed the preceding considerations in order to place in its proper context the *modus operandi* of the champion of observation — what I was fifteen years ago. We will see in this chapter how he expresses himself and how he used to express himself. And we will study — as I study him, and myself — to what extent and in what context the abstract argumentation of the apologists and rebels (of whom I used to be one) preserves an element of truth. Set in the progress of a dialectic evolution, this chapter of explanation and refutation is not without interest: It constitutes (as we shall see at the end of the book) a personal testimony.

The Dialogue of Evil and Morality

Morals are an expression of man's effort to adapt himself to the alien presence of evil in this world. It would be impossible to try to understand the one without the other.

The scandal — or the mystery — of evil will always shock the human conscience, which confronts it with the most troubled justifications, so troubled, in fact, that they sometimes overflow into non-justification and consecrate evil as taboo. Such a levy of arguments makes a disturbing spectacle, all shields thrown up against the plague from God. I know of nothing more pitiful than the great haste to conceal evil behind defensive arguments (which would be enough, were there nothing else, to make it into an accused defendant). Nothing is more pitiful than man's cowardice, his complicity with evil. There is no way to disguise evil — so let us look it in the eye. Some revolts are more edifying than any apology. But then we must ask ourselves what our attitude will be in the face of evil: *What,* in other words, *will be our set of morals?*

It would be impossible for us to speak of the evil committed by man without having considered the problem of evil in general: The two categories overlap, and moral evil can only be defined against a background of metaphysical guilt or innocence. In both cases evil is real only because of man; without him, the universe is neutral.

But what is evil, that we should speak of it in such terms? Certainly it is not an entity, but an experience: a whole collection of bad experiences, imperfections, and pains, everything that shocks our conscience and is in disharmony with this creation which should, it would seem, be good if it is true that it came from the hands of a perfect Creator.

Two attitudes appear to be possible in the face of evil: acceptance or refusal. Without faith, there is only one: refusal. Its history is that of human revolt with its two faces — two enemy brothers, individualistic nihilism and totalitarian nihilism. Perhaps there is a way through and beyond rebellion (as attacking soldiers must jump over fallen bodies) which leads to reconciliation with the world. Any morality is transcendent, a form of asceticism. Any ascetic effort reaches the goal of this reconciliation if it pushes far and hard enough. All moralities, without an exception, even those of pleasure, of self-interest, or of pride, come together in their culmination of love, providing only that they follow their own rules to their logical conclusions. The culmination of ascetic effort is love, but love has meaning only when gained through ascetic effort.

Evil and Human Freedom

Some counter evil by arguing that it is a nonexistent problem, others in the name of man's "free will."

Human freedom in evil is called sin. A whole set of explanations for evil are structured by reference to sin and its consequences.

God could not have permitted evil unless we deserved it somehow or other. So goes the myth of original sin. Evil has been in the world [1] and in us since the sin of Adam (man), as a kind of punishment or fall which our ancestor earned for us. It is of little importance here whether this guilt belonged to a specific ancestor

[1] "We must be guilty in order to exculpate God," writes Groethuysen in *Origines de l'esprit bourgeois en France* [Origins of the bourgeois spirit in France], p. 135. Let us remark that the scandal of suffering in animals (sinless creatures) is imputed, as is the totality of the world's woe, to man's sin.

or whether Adam symbolizes man's guilt in general. Neither is it my task to study the dogma of original sin in either of its forms, as hereditary guilt or as a simple hereditary fall. Evil has less to do with the transmissibility of sin than with its existence from the very beginning.

What is, in fact, incomprehensible is how man, before the existence of evil, could have committed the first sin.[2] And it is not the original sin which can explain evil since it had need itself of evil in order to have been possible.[3]

The reply comes back that if evil did exist before sin, it was only as a theoretical possibility included in divine infinity. And *God wanted man to be free, and if free, capable of choosing evil.* Only liberty (pure and "indifferent" in Adam, but soiled with concupiscence in his descendants) was able to give evil any reality in the universe. Evdokimov writes:

> If there is no place in God for evil, there is nonetheless in him an absolute knowledge of its possibility, since God is absolute fullness. . . . Starting with the idea of God, we can reach the idea of evil; we can at least imagine it. The freedom of the created being extracts this idea from nothingness and introduces it in its own right. This passage from idea to existence (analogous to the ontological argument) is the very essence of the creative act. . . . The creature, for a moment, has become God, the creature created evil. . . .[4]

This reasoning runs into two decisive difficulties:

1. The idea, the "possibility" of evil is not inherent in divine infinity.

2. The possibility of choosing evil is by no means indispensable for human liberty.

The first point deserves little of our time: Divine infinity, or divine fullness, as you prefer, only implies the idea or the possibility of evil if this idea or possibility has already (beforehand) been

[2] A well-known difficulty, hundreds of times expressed: "We are sinners because of the sin of our first ancestor; but our first ancestor, why was he a sinner?" wrote J. J. Rousseau in *Lettre à Christophe de Beaumond,* archbishop of Paris. "Original sin explains everything but its own principle." Cf. also the same objection taken from St. de Guaita, *Essais des sciences maudites* [Essays on the occult sciences], quoted by Evdokimov, *Dostoïevski et le problème du mal* [Dostoevski and the problem of evil], p. 248. The same idea is found in A. France, *Les dieux ont soif* [Thirst of the gods].

[3] Divine punishment seems, moreover, to have changed nothing in our condition, and we have no reason to envy the so-called happy innocence of the earthly Paradise. I would not say that man was happy there; he met his greatest woe there. Neither would I say that there he accomplished good in a permanent state of grace; there he committed the greatest evil. So it was possible there for him to commit evil at every step. He had in him, before sin, the seeds of all his errors, all his pains; and this seed was really only waiting for the best occasion to put all its virtuality into action.

[4] Evdokimov, *op. cit.,* pp. 154, 168.

posed. And the very existence of this possibility is contingent: *It exists only to the extent that God wanted it to exist.*

The possibility of evil seems all the more difficult to accept in God because it is so incompatible with the infinite perfection which we attribute to him. Evil is imperfection; perfection excludes it. In order for absolute goodness to think evil, it must no longer be itself. Alleging that we are not dealing with real evil but with possible evil changes nothing. The idea of possible evil is enough to put an irrevocable mark on complete goodness (as does the idea of possible adultery, according to the gospel). The sole idea of nothingness "as an ideal assertion" already contains the seed of nothingness. If man's only role is to realize (actualize) an evil already present in God, the veritable creative act of evil hardly belongs to him; it belongs to God.

The second point will require a more extensive examination. It seems very difficult to forget the idea that the exercise of liberty necessarily includes the possibility of choice between good and bad and that man's liberty made him liable to a choice of evil.[5] Is removing the power of refusing good, removing the possibility of evil, not doing away with liberty? *Evil indispensable for the exercise of freedom; evil explained by sin* (sinful liberty): these are two forms of the same thesis which, we must carefully note, put the full blame on human initiative – evil is thus the result of committed evil; universal catastrophes are the result of human responsibility.

It would be too easy to emphasize the inhuman quality of such an "imputation," and it would speak only to the heart. To reach the intelligence, I would have to show the logical difficulties of a hypothesis which makes evil dependent on liberty and its practice.

It is strange that most thinkers refuse to consider a world deprived of evil without seeing it as necessarily without freedom. Thus, due to their standpoint, they commit the error of preserving the "memory" of a possible evil which they do not want to lose. And it is just this presupposition which is in doubt. The possibility of evil is only a part of our freedom to the extent that God desired and drew from nothingness that possibility which thereby became open to man.

Here, as with the raw fact of the painfulness of pain,[6] we must

[5] "Is evil not the offspring of good, necessary for created man to be free. . . ? Is the kingdom of liberty possible without the direct experience of knowing evil?" (Evdokimov, *op. cit.*, pp. 151–153). Cf., for example, J. Chevalier, "Le sens du péché" [The meaning of sin] in *L'Homme et le péché* [Man and sin], collectively authored and published in *Présences* (Paris: Librairie Plon). This opinion is one of the most widespread.

[6] Cf. p. 89.

avoid concluding that a factual situation implies a rightful necessity. The fact that the choice of evil is an undeniable part of our world and of our liberty (let us take this for granted without going into the new problems it poses) does not mean that it *had* to play this role.

So we must accept, I repeat, that many confuse liberty with the power of opposites, the "indifferent" choice between one hand and the other, between good and evil. Another study would be necessary to examine this fundamental problem properly.[7] May I simply plead here in favor of that liberty which is much more genuine than an indifferent power of choice: that which is accomplished by the acceptance of truth and goodness, with no possible refusal. It is yet to be proved, some say, that God is free, that he can only desire good! This is giving to the saints a freedom of choice which the impenitent defenders of free will would consider "deprived" of the indispensable possibility of evil!

If good were always to win every battle, if evil were ever excluded, would there be any room for a choice? If God's proofs were always conclusive, would the fact of *believing,* the act of faith, the act of freedom, not be degraded to simple knowledge? Thus what is tragically called "God's silence," like evil, becomes for many apologists the basis and condition *sine qua non* of human *liberty.* This opinion has always deeply shocked me.

God keeps silence, you say, hides himself,[8] *in order that* we might seek him out and go to him through our own effort, our own movement, initiative, and liberty. If he manifested himself, our adhesion, our faith, and our love would be as automatic as iron falling to earth. It would be a violence excluding all liberty. But distance in time and space enables us to measure more accurately

[7] I have studied it, for example, in *Etudes philosophiques,* no. 2 (1950), "De la liberté chez Descartes" [Liberty in Descartes' writings], and no. 3 (1952) "Le problème du refus" [The Problem of Refusal].

[8] Those who speak of "God's silence" take care not to speak of a total silence (which would do away with the problem); more troubling in their eyes is a half-silence, the blend of clearness and obscurity which, like the contradictory stimuli applied to Pavlov's dogs, incites confusion and neurosis. Yes/No is worse than no. It is said that the infinite God shows himself perhaps, but seldom, insufficiently, by no means superabundantly and infinitely, as would seem to be proper for infiniteness. This doubtful presence, hardly certain, subject to eclipse, satisfies neither our thirst nor its own nature. And it is, in fact, easy to answer that it is our blindness which makes God's presence of little importance. God is not silent; he has spoken to us, is speaking to us, and is present every moment for the one who knows how to see and listen. "Listen, O Israel." The "silence of God" is scaled to our refusal, which finds it easier to change its name! Contesting the objectivity of this silence undoubtedly turns the problem inside out.

the space of our initiative and enables us also not to stop the "suspense" which includes not only our separation from God, but also our return to him.

It seems rather equivocal to me to claim that our liberty depends on the obscurity of the conditions under which it is exercised. Is the essence of liberty not to manifest itself obviously whenever the means are granted it to manifest itself — in complete freedom? Since Descartes the same confusion has often been repeated between "indifference" which is a weakness and that which is a power.[9] What an attack on our liberty is this removal of possibilities of choice brought on by "God's silence"! Furthermore, it would be insinuating that liberty is scaled to the negative conditions in which it is exercised. Does this mean that the Australians, to whom God manifested himself *less* than to the Israelites, were freer to choose him? The least that we can say is that it would be hazardous to claim that our liberty is dependent on a lesser manifestation of God! Liberty is exercised in everyone, according to his place in society and his personal situation: the Chinese and the European, the believer and the unbeliever, the apostle of Christ's time or the twentieth-century astronaut. Is it not childish to claim that this liberty would be defectively expressed or even annulled in that man to whom God would manifest himself *totally*?[10] Yes, accepting that liberty is truly exercised only in relative ignorance, in "the silence of God," is, in reality, a monstrosity. And the same is true of the allegation that liberty depends on the provisions for evil spread out in a well-assorted display of choices!

Moreover — and let us close here the discussion of evil as related to liberty — some may endeavor to associate original goodness and liberty *(with the possibility for this liberty,* accepted hypothetically only, *to choose evil),* but evil will never be chosen. And if it is true that man was created free and good (without sinful desires and without temptations, since both presuppose that evil which must be excluded from man's original nature), is it possible for a good and free being to commit the evil which some would have him able to choose? It is obvious that *liberty could not choose evil unless evil were already dwelling in the person exercising that liberty.*

[9] Cf. Jacques Sarano, *Etudes philosophiques,* no. 2 (1950), pp. 213 ff.

[10] Would this be depriving of his liberty anyone who was a direct witness to Christ's life? What about Thomas, who touched his wounds? In fact, the actual, bodily presence of Christ under Pontius Pilate was probably as much of an obstacle as a help. And the way a contemporary of Christ received him determined whether or not that man was a direct witness.

So evil was not created by our liberty, neither was it indispensable for the exercise of liberty. Free will only solves the mystery of evil if we consent to leave the enigma without an answer and if the impossibility of finding a solution is accepted as a (hidden) solution. The problem of the creation of evil may, therefore, not be considered only on the level of divinity, before sin[11] (if we may properly use the word "before" – this type of priority has little to do with time).

Was Evil Necessary for the Divine Economy?

Is this a Manichaean solution? But unless we think of a powerless and finite God, could evil exist outside of him, against him, as a rival, an autonomous power causing him to fail?

In the West we usually reject this hypothesis and choose the opposite, which supposes evil to be a kind of servant of good.

Evil is seen as a factor in progress, in transcending self, and a condition for the greatest good – a paradoxical finality which at first sight revolts our conscience. How could evil, the servant of good, ever offend God? (But God is able to transform even the offense against himself into a good.) Above all, is the detour through evil admissible in Him who is able immediately to give the best? If the good obtained by evil is "better," why did he arrange things so that good could only become better at the price of evil? Pain is a strengthening trial for one, debilitating and disastrous for another – its results follow the situation and the resources of the individual. The notions of merit, difficulties vanquished, and victorious joy, are only expressions of the advantages man was able to extract from evil, not a justification of evil.

Evil can both serve and retard progress. Progress, in turn, *denies* the state that it modifies without thereby expressing an evil. Need, fruitful dissatisfaction, and generating progress may not be identified with pain.

Some have emphasized the *dialectic* relationship which binds together production and destruction. Man's *negativistic* action is both destructive and creative. Man "creates by destroying nature, the world, a world which did not exist. . . ." [12] Nothingness eats away

[11] The most competent theologians no longer count on committed evil (sin, and more particularly original sin) to explain evil. Cf. R. P. Sertilanges, *Le problème du mal* [The problem of evil] (Paris: Aubier-Montaigne, 1951), vol. 2, p. 25.

[12] "Etudes hégéliennes," in *Deucalion,* 5 (October, 1955), Neuchâtel: la Baconnière, p. 23. Georges Bataille, *Hegel, la mort et le sacrifice* [Hegel, death and sacrifice].

at man's world; man's action gnaws away at nature, which is both a dream and beauty. Man is specifically destructive; there are in him possibilities of death, of death desired and played out in spite of life. Such is the force of its negativeness. By a voluntary death, by agreeing to risk his life, man creates himself as man. Man is the very image of the destructive negativeness of death. What a paradox: This negativeness is a worker; it engenders the work which transforms the world and cooperates with God's work.

Elsewhere I have attempted to outline the relationship between the work of destruction and the work of creation.[13] It is certain that the destructive act first reveals phenomenologically a discord between man and the object, a discord which we may describe as being out of phase.

It is only by a patient job of *relativizing* the destructive act — which would attempt to see in it a defect or, on the contrary, a transcending of the original meaning of an object — that we may perhaps venture as far as the region of absolute destruction.

The mysterious nucleus of wickedness, of destructive desire, of the free refusal of being, of evil freely committed, or of sin is the place where the effort to understand must finally yield to judgment, where certain motivations are taken from their original psychological or empirical plan and invested with a metaphysical meaning that involves our liberty. Hence, pride is seen as a desire for power.

On the phenomenological level, destruction might have been included in the idea of a discord in which man and his work are out of phase — with works falling behind man, or with man falling behind and destroying the object. But on the metaphysical level, the opposing pair, misunderstanding/recognition, gives way to the mysterious pair, wickedness/love.[14]

Here we see the limit which very literally forms an impassable wall for the tragic conception of the world founded on the Hegelian negation, or rather on the Nietzschean (or Sivaite) "Die and Become." Of course, creation through destruction, the production of better through evil, could provide us with a key for the understanding of our developing world. But this vision of a universe re-creating itself and building progress on its own ruins may not be distinguished from the hell of an eternal return in which creative destruction is only confused with absolute destruction by

[13] J. Sarano, *L'homme et ses oeuvres* [Man and his works], actes du IXe Congrès des sociétés de philosophie de langue française (Paris: Presses Universitaires de France, 1957), no. 3 in the series *Etudes philosophiques,* p. 60.

[14] *Ibid.,* p. 62.

one who accepts that evil is a useful servant in the edification of good – evil understood as pain and slaughter, life feeding on death at every level of the vegetable and animal kingdoms.

Yes, evil can be relativized, brought to the human level, by man's demand for that amelioration of which it is an evidence and, using a figure of speech, onto which it is grafted. In the case of pure passivity there is no evil. It only means a vague contrast of good, the spur, the thorn which it plants in man's flesh. Is evil only a shadow, the power behind the throne of good?[15]

Evil Without an Autonomous Existence: Relative to Good and a Parasite of Being

Slowly but surely we are working toward those theories which go so far as to deny any real consistency to evil. What is evil, if not the negative for, and the proof of, our calling for good?

Evil is a "nothing" grafted on the only being: good. For evil is a non-being, its only form is that of a parasite of good.

Evil, a loss of goodness – who would deny it? But as a loss of or an obstacle to good, a parasite, it is inevitably a defect. Its relation to good makes its painful weight of flesh and blood no less of a reality for all living beings.

[15] In Blondel's thought we find suffering and evil presented as being in man the proof of a superior ambition and superior calling (*L'Action,* 1893, pp. 33, 35, 38, 154; on suffering, pp. 328, 380 ff.; on evil, p. 334). A development of evil understood as a condition for good may be found in Roger Verneaux, *Problèmes et mysteres du mal* [Problems and Mysteries of Evil], (Paris: La Colombe, 1956), for example, pp. 62, 63, 82. But the same author, e.g., p. 141 of the same book, calls to mind that "it is never legitimate to accomplish evil in order to attain a good result." However, "We assert, not that evil effectively works for the good of the universe, but that the idea itself has nothing absurd or even unlikely about it" (p. 62). Again: "The evil that he [God] permits to exist within his work is itself an instrument of good" (p. 82). Finally, here is a justification for evil which goes back to the disciple Thomas: "Why is it proper for certain beings to be corruptible? Because otherwise there would be lacking in the universe that degree of perfection and goodness which material beings represent" (p. 95). *It was proper,* we are assured, for the world to contain a multiplicity of beings (p. 94) and for carnivores to be surrounded by other animals for them to devour (p. 81)! I, for my part, have trouble believing this. Has our author not confused finiteness and evil (pp. 79, 80, 95)? And is there not a dubious distinction between God's *will* for evil and his *permission?*

Nabert's approach is entirely different, as we shall see a bit later, for example, in his treatment of those evils "which appear to us as the condition of a greater good." See *Essai sur le mal* [A Study of Evil] (Paris: Presses Universitaires de France, 1955), p. 29. Against the confusion between finiteness and evil, cf. pp. 34 ff. P. Ricoeur has written some fine pages on finiteness as a *disproportion* between the finite and the infinite, the source of the undifferentiated pathos of misery (evil), the common trunk from which committed and suffered evil sprout. See P. Ricoeur, *Finitude et culpabilité* [Finiteness and Guilt] (Paris: Aubier-Montaigne), vol. 1, chapter 1.

We must, first of all, avoid the all too frequent confusion between *a loss of goodness* and the *finiteness* inherent in every creature. Saying that evil is the inevitable corollary of our imperfection or finiteness as created beings is really turning the question around and disguising evil as a *"lesser good,"* and it is therefore according evil a *"certain degree of participation in goodness,"* in other words, more or less of a good in its period of formation, its preparation.

We find this to be a facile sophism. Considering evil as a ransom, the very sign of our slow climb, of our painful ascension toward goodness, is forgetting that a lesser good (a degree of goodness, no matter how small) is never an evil, that evil is rather a reversed good, a good whose sign or whose pole has been changed. By no means is it a small segment of the same vector, but a vector turned in the opposite direction. Evil turns its back on good, is the destruction of meaning, fraudulent deprivation of meaning, the refusal of good (by man or by the cosmos, one or the other).

We must also note that sweetening evil by hiding it under the cloak of goodness-not-yet-realized (or perhaps only imperfect, as with any created, finite good) is no way of reconciling it with the tragedy of committed evil, sin itself. Neither finiteness nor sin can explain evil, since each of these terms points out the insufficiency of the other. Finiteness, for its part, is no more successful in explaining the presence of sin than that of pain. Sin implies more than a lack of power (if we mean to take sin into account in the study of evil and pain). It presupposes something else, in fact, the very opposite: a *power,* that of refusal. Of course, sin is servitude, a defective state. But it is one that has been chosen and taken over by a power. Sin is therefore the paradox of powerlessness borne by a power; it is the very paradox of liberty (in evil).[16] It is certain that this powerlessness which is a power is open to controversy, but here I wish only to emphasize that a refusal, a turning of the back on evil, may not be accommodated with evil reduced to a vaguely inferior degree of goodness.

Man is less perfect because he is a creature: but a lesser perfec-

[16] I emphasized this paradox between "a lack in the form of a refusal, non-liberty in the form of an act of liberty, and my non-act in the form of an act" in several comments I made on *Le volontaire et l'involontaire* [Voluntary and involuntary] by P. Ricoeur (cf. *Etudes philosophiques,* no. 4, 1955): "I make myself a slave," writes P. Ricoeur, "I impute myself with the fault which takes away my empire over myself" (p. 29). Is this not admitting, willingly or not, that the lack is taken over by a power? Is it not making a lack into a power since it has to be chosen? Choice means power. Asserting that a weakness has been chosen is making of it a strength! It is reversing the poles and making a lack into a refusal!

tion is not subjection to evil; even less is it to choose evil. An inferior degree of perfection is not opposition to perfection. Evil means opposition, reversal, and is in no wise a part of the law of growth for created beings, no matter how imperfect they are.

The idea alone of *deprivation,* without going as far as the double refusal implied in error, is something other than finiteness: (1) because it constitutes a lack; (2) because it is felt to be such. Not only a lack *of* something, but a painful lack – not only the objective fact which makes it evil, but the fact that it is suffered as a deprivation – is the double meaning of the word "lack."

I am deprived of seeing ultraviolet rays, but in no way do I consider this deprivation to be an evil. It is doubtlessly an imperfection and can be chalked up to my finite nature. It is no evil to be natural, to live out one's nature. Living according to one's nature and accomplishing it can be a good – happiness, perfection in its own way, harmony in order. On the other hand, being deprived of sight, blindness by injury or from birth, is a deprivation in the true sense of the word, a violence inflicted on my nature, by no stretch of the imagination an imperfection inherent to my nature – although the first type of privation can lead to the second. *My nature is* such that my eye can be put out, my child can be born an idiot or deformed if his mother had a certain kind of measles during pregnancy.

Now I am making common reference to the notions of one's nature open to discussion, and of anomalies or dispositions that run *counter to nature,* and so we return to the irreducible experience of *pain* (a deprivation felt as such). I should make myself more clear.

Anomaly: It is "abnormal" for me to be lame, hunchbacked, or blind, but it is "normal" not to be able to run as fast as an elephant. I purposely yielded to the temptation of using the equivocal terms of "normal" and "abnormal," which may refer to no serious criterion on the order of being, but which require a subjective preference and a disproportion between demand and possibility. It is both normal that I cannot run as fast as Tom or Dick (considering the inequality of individuals) and abnormal (considering what I would like to have expected of myself). That is why anomaly has no meaning if it may not be referred to and upheld by its subjective counterpart, the pain of suffering that anomaly.

So here again it is pain itself which poses the problem, and we refer the reader to the first part of the book: Pain here has the meaning of a deprivation felt to be such. The theologians are free to find abnormal the opposite possibility, that of "playing a beautiful tune to warn a man that he is going to burn himself."[17] For in truth there is nothing to keep a warning of danger from being nonpainful. (The sight of a car bearing down on me makes me jump aside; in this case the rapidity and specificity of the sensory warning had no need of pain. But these considerations were sufficiently developed in Part One for us not to have to come back to them again; their place here would be as answers to the apologists' arguments.) Pain as such, whatever its mysterious ways may be, even if it were created for the better, is no less unjustifiable. Why choose the painful way to obtain a higher good? We must not take a contingent fact for a rightful necessity — this we have already seen.

But the equivocal notions of "normal" and "abnormal" are expressions of a *relation* rather than of a fact. Pain and grief are born of a *disproportion* between what we have and what we would have liked to have had. So man suffocates in his "normal" human condition (finite, imperfect).

Evil and Disproportion

Here pain acquires another face: It is man's very demands for progress toward infinity which make him unhappy; and this unhappiness is added on to direct pain itself, the injuries and griefs which we designate *stricto sensu* by the word "pain." It is this inequality between our aspirations and our powerlessness which nourishes the attitudes of a Prometheus, on the one hand, and of his enemies, on the other: man's pride and the desire, legitimate for one, illegitimate for the other, of eating from the tree of knowledge or of life. Guilty or not, illegitimate or not, man's inner demands are imperious, a source of pain, for they run into the wall of failure, of death, of impossibility, and of powerlessness. This is where "normal" becomes "abnormal"; "natural" is transformed into "anti-natural"; and *it is no longer enough* to say that our limits and our evils "are definitely subject to the laws of nature."[18] Here we witness the ground of our problem shifting, and this shift is worthy of our attention. Earlier I called to mind a commonsense distinction. I suffer from being one-eyed, deprived of one eye, but I do not suffer at all from not possessing a thousand pairs of eyes. What is not a part of my nature is not a painful deprivation for me, but what amputates and mutilates my nature is painful. I

[17] R. P. Sertilanges, *op. cit.*, vol. 2, p. 15.

[18] J. Nabert, *op. cit.*, chapter 1, p. 3. A bit later I will take up several points found in this important study.

added that this distinction disappears whenever the possibility of amputation or mutilation *belongs* to the very nature of my organs. But the same distinction disappears by the opposite consideration: not possessing a thousand eyes or immortality *becomes* pain through the intervention of man's inner desires which accept no limits, and by comparison to the infinite dimensions of the human thirst for infiniteness. Is it not useless to note that "evil" only exists through our exorbitant pretensions – that this "evil" can therefore claim no reality in the proper sense of the term, that it is "nothing" except the shadow cast by human ambition, certainly a sign of his greatness in the image of God, but also of the fact that he is a spoiled child too hasty to touch his inheritance? Yes, what use is it to *shift* evil around, to take it from objects in order to settle it in some other illness, an illness inherent to his very nature, his divine calling, and his yearning for infiniteness? "Normal" is entirely swallowed up in "abnormal," for man is out of balance with his own nature; he is not what he is and his finiteness is frustration. His imperfection contains the worm of pain which is eating out his heart. Hence it is impossible to claim that some item belongs to our nature and another not, since our nature *is not*.[19]

We must return to Nabert's fundamental question: What is our criterion for judging evil as "unjustifiable"? [20] Is a revolt against facts, risen from our sensitivity, enough of a basis for a legal condemnation?

"What is necessary," asks Nabert, "in order for this (condemnation) to cease being arbitrary, since it is included neither in the categories of speculative reason, nor in the must-be of morality? Nothing less is necessary than an act *within the assertion itself which includes its own guarantee of itself,* and which brings to light at the same time an absolute opposition between the pure spirituality to which it bears witness and the structure of the world." [21]

In other words, as I see it, we have no obligation to give reasons

[19] That healthy philosophy which counsels me to be satisfied with the natural order of things is no longer current today. The class struggle is, in its own way, evidence of the evolution to be observed in the notion of what is natural (or normal). A given miserable class was not "miserable" as long as it thought its condition to be "natural" or "normal." Its realization of its own status as a class is identical with its unhappiness and the "abnormal" misery of that very same condition—in fact, it doubles that misery. In this way evil can be found either in the condition itself or in the realization that the condition is intolerable.

[20] Cf. Nabert, *op. cit.*, pp. 3, 19, 23, 25, 28–31.

[21] *Ibid.*, p. 31 (italics ours).

for our condemnation of a given structure of the world, or of its total structure, for such a condemnation is itself its own proof. A revolt, in fact, is *equivalent* to a legal revolt, and this by a very particular short circuit which I am about to explain.

At the very moment when I demand of an actual revolt (that is, a revolt based on our sensitivity) its right to judge an "evil" as being evil, this very revolt is a fact and a reality and so constitutes itself a flagrant crime of the same nature as what it is proclaiming. It is its own best witness; being unjustifiable, it is added to the unjustifiability of evil, is enough to ensure that there is an unjustifiability of evil, and is enough to ensure that it is itself justifiable. In this way, if the unjustifiability of evil is contested in an object, it is shifted to the revolt itself, that illness (that evil) of human sensibility. This is what I call a short circuit: The factual revolt engenders its own right—it is the relay of a first evil which incited it and brought it forth as a second evil.

What right have we to condemn? The notion of condemnation contains its own justification, not in its specific content, but in its general form. If this factual revolt were reduced to its basic reality, it could not be considered in the form of a judgment.

Were we to suppose that a condemnation is not justifiable in a given case (although there are very few which give us any reason for uncertainty), it could still not be contested in every case without thereby denying its very meaning as a condemnation; it would become an empty word, *flatus vocis*. Now, the condemnation (that is, the very notion of evil) *does* exist. It necessarily has its own content (it is the condemnation of something), without which it would cancel itself out or would never have been born. The condemnation could not exist without that which is condemned.

Let us state this case in other terms: It is impossible to *reduce* condemnation/judgment to a revolt of fact (a simple biological reaction) for the simple reason that we do not confuse them. We clearly distinguish the difference between the two, and this difference proves the specificity of the terms which it enables us to differentiate. In just the same way, the sceptic does not wear himself out trying to persuade us that he is telling the truth without thereby showing himself to be wrong. The rationalist (or scientist) does not wear himself out trying to reduce thought to a molecular combination without thereby forgetting that his faith in science, in reason, is what makes the very conclusion he is seeking impossible. There are contestations which prove the very point they are contesting, because they agreed to discuss the subject. So it is with legal condemnation, the renewal and the ratification of our sensitivity and its reaction.

The content of a particular judgment sends me on to the justification of judgment in general. But I notice that the latter is justified by its own existence. The act of condemning something generates the reality (of the truth) of its general content – evil. The notion of condemnation implies an evil (if only by missing its goal and mistaking its object). I would say that *revolt/ condemnation* (or judgment) / *evil* present three faces of a single reality, each of which is sufficient to prove the other two.

Evil, a False or Partial Judgment

The preceding considerations should be enough, we would think, to convince those apologists who attempt a sort of dissolution of evil in illusion. Some claim that *we only see evil!* Others claim that "the world is not necessarily ordered according to human finality."

God, they both say, does not necessarily act in accordance with the demands of our *limited consciousness.* So our consciousness was given to limit us! Nothing reaches us except through our consciousness: Declaring that it is worthless is taking from it every means of discerning and loving good; it is probably annihilating it. Neither good, evil, nor God have any meaning in such a case.

But does a finite being have the right to pass judgment on everything, of which it represents only the minutest part? "How could it be that a part know the whole?" asked Pascal. The Book of Job recounts the same mortification of "righteousness" faced with "unjustifiability." Such a critique throws doubt on the very possibility for our human mind to appreciate the meaning of the universe.[22]

Refusing us the right to examine God's plans would be stopping our study before it started. Evil would only be an appearance due to our feeble judgment: an optical illusion![23] But reducing evil to

[22] How can creation be condemned without including my judgment which is a part of it? This is a sophism. For if it is said that in a defective universe my judgment which condemns it is also defective, or if it is said that the universe is good, the perversion of my judgment would be enough to contest that goodness.

[23] "All that is left is to consider evil as an illusion, an appearance of being, behind which is to be found the genuine reality: goodness" (Evdokimov, *op. cit.,* p. 316). Gandhi: "If the intimate thoughts of the creator were known to us, we would discover the place which belongs even to harmful beings in creation." Gandhi, *Le jeune Inde* [Young India] (Paris: Editions Stock), p. 32. "The reason for evil is only to be found in good," writes an author commenting on the disciple Thomas, "for all was designed for good; if we do not see that good, it is because we are *in the wrong position* (italics mine) to see it. . . ."

a subjective illusion on man's part is just pushing the difficulty back a notch without solving it. Saying that evil is not in the world, but in the way we understand it, is only removing it from one place and putting it in another. It will still be there – if only in the idea we have of the world. If evil did not exist, how could we see it, unless it were because of some defect which would itself be an evil?

But there is no retreat. The illusion of evil is itself an evil only for the human mind, which must therefore be limited. But "limited" is not enough, since my lack of comprehension is negatively expressed by the idea of evil. We should be saying "corrupted," and evil is a part of the corruption! It is obvious that the two partners could keep the ball going back and forth indefinitely – if it were not rather easy for common sense to put an end to it by the consideration that, after all, we are all inescapably dwelling within the limits of human consciousness. The same is true for both the one who contests the worth of what that consciousness teaches and for him who accepts it.[24]

[24] It has been correctly said that the essence of reason is to know its place and proper limits. But this is still reason talking and it has thus placed itself outside the limits which it recognized as proper for reason. This is what we could call a "constituting" consciousness, "outside the standard of consciousness," Nabert would say, and this is what some would like to take away from us—and from themselves. Sooner or later the person who judges that we are incapable of judging ourselves must take heed to his own judgment. Asserting that our mind cannot understand the meaning of "evil" is just one opinion of that mind. *Proclaiming as a true idea that our mind is deluding itself is the very denial of the idea itself.—Nota bene* 1: What does the phrase, "If God exists, he must be incomprehensible," mean? Obviously, God can only be incomprehensible because of the very comprehensible idea that we have of God (eternal and temporal, perfect creator of an imperfect creation). Some emphasize the *heterogeneity of what divinity requires of the human consciousness.* It should not astonish or revolt us that this fact astonishes us and revolts us. It should, in fact, appear to be the rule to anyone who has reflected on divine incommensurability (cf. the examples of Abraham and Job as illuminated by Kierkegaard). So I believe that God is love, but I do not understand how—and to do so I would go so far as to believe, as to see my own thoughts blown to shreds before absurdity—a loving God permits or requires that the worst evil come about! But we must beware of the subjective, even pathological, nature of my blind surrender! This also is a prejudice which I must yet study. Instead of saying that God is incomprehensible, let us say that my faith requires him to be so. I forego all coherency because of the strength and the virtue of my faith. Faith is permitted everything, but I must at least be warned that *I am putting into my faith a part of myself* and so must be wary of the qualities I am thus interjecting.

Placing God beyond what is imaginable is another way of imagining him. The term, an "incomprehensible" God, risks being mostly of literary value: it is *meaningful* of divine infinitude; it is no excuse for evil, nor may it be used to invoke a hypothetical mission of evil.

Nota bene 2: Saying that evil is a mystery is saying that it is incompatible

We would, however, be wrong if we retained nothing from this confrontation but the memory of extreme formulations. It is true that many trials and "anomalies" which appear to us to be intolerable in the rush of a first attack become "normal" after reflection. Did we perhaps not know how to consider them? Would a wider and more penetrating vision be able to understand what now shocks us; could it account for evil, absorb it, as it were? Partially, perhaps, but variations of content or of percentage have a very relative effect on the problem of the *existence* of evil ("one single child in agony . . ."). Yes, the unjustifiable pain of a small child will eternally give flat contradiction to those who say, "Look closer." Perhaps a superhuman understanding would discern with Leibnitz the "sufficient reason" for everything in this world which, although it is not the best of all possible worlds for us, still must be made just that, through the "smallest possible amount of evil." [25] Our "incomprehension," our painful astonishment before the pain of a small child, stays on, and we oscillate between the evil of this painful incomprehension itself and the raw, irreducible, immediate pain to which it harks back, which seemed to weigh heavy on the entire first part of this book devoted to pain.

Pain being what it is, we would make of it an evil only by a faulty judgment — just as our sensations are mistaken in their perception of the real dimensions of the sun. The intervention of reason enables me to back off from my affective or sensory partiality and to judge objectively that I am a poor judge: I cannot grasp the totality of the problem (of creation) with my eyes. My reason *frees itself from itself, as it were, by recognizing its own limits.* It becomes partial by the definition of that partiality which is due to our finiteness. Evil is swallowed up by a false judgment, or

---

with a perfect God. It is not, therefore, protecting oneself from an assertion but rather becoming compromised in it and asserting, by way of a detour, that the speaker wants to have nothing to do with the postulate of a perfect God. Pretending that the problem of evil is unsolvable is imposing on us (while all the time saying the contrary) a solution for the problem of evil—a tendentious solution, for under the term "mystery" the only aim is to camouflage and justify evil. Of course, evil is a mystery; otherwise it would not merit all the ruckus it has caused. But when we say mystery we mean that the revolt on the one hand be respected just as much as the surrender or unshakable confidence on the other. Mystery does not mean absolution. We must not place too cheap a price on human protest. From Kirilov to Camus it has itself been a way of speaking of mystery (1952).

[25] God "could not do otherwise," some apologists say (cf., for example, Verneaux, *op. cit.*, p. 81). "He permitted the least amount of evil possible in a creation such as he conceived it" (p. 83), they add (although Verneaux does not adopt the argument for his own use) and think they are thereby adding to God's omnipotence!

rather, *it corresponds to a judgment which is correct on one plane, false on another;* all that is necessary is for it to be properly aligned. Evil only remains revolting, only remains evil, by the ignorance of our ignorance, an ignorance which bounds from man to man, bounces down step after step as far as the eye can see. It is complete blindness, an absolute refusal to understand, which considers itself to be a proof.

No! That is not enough. Claiming that blindness rectifies the situation does not finish the tragedy. It only emasculates it; it closes our eyes against precise, positive realities which do not give us the leisure of being suspended between an absurd evil and a providential evil. The two pans of the balance are not equal. Pain is an exceptionally privileged, but glaring, crime on the list of the world's absurdities. If there is partiality, it also is flagrant, just as foolish for the defense as for the prosecution. It is not enough to *detach* oneself from oneself in order to justify and evaporate the world's pain into thin air. *Restoration,* if necessary, is necessary on both sides. A simple avowal of ignorance is not enough to save evil, neither is an effort to be impartial. But a *partiality* just as passionate, just as risky, and even more absurd than revolt, can save a very compromised battle. I am not moving up from partiality to impartiality to objectivity. A detached attitude is not enough to qualify one as a judge. We must give up a lot in order to become reconciled with pain, with evil. We must be ready to lay down a tremendous initial investment and grant a great deal of credit to creation and the creator.

Evil: An Irreducible Reality, but It Requires that We Grant the Creator a Great Deal of Credit

It is with this idea of credit that I would like to close this chapter, for it seems to me both to sum up the vanity of the explanations for evil,[26] and to launch the act of testimony which constitutes the

[26] Here is what Kant had to say about the vanity of explaining evil: "Job's friends accepted the doctrine that considers all the world's evils as explainable by divine justice. . . . But Job protested vehemently that his conscience going back over all his life could find no fault, and as for those errors unavoidable because of human fragility, God himself knew well that he had created him fallible. He declared himself in favor of the theory of God's pure and simple will: 'God is one,' he said, 'and does what he wants. . . .' And if we consider these two theories, it is probable that the friends' hypothesis would appear from a speculative point of view to be more reasonable and more marked with religious humility. And if Job had appeared before some tribunal of theologians . . . he would by all appearances have been in a very bad position. Thus,

investment I mentioned a moment ago and which I will study in detail in chapters 3 and 4.

It is useless to fight the positive *reality* of evil. Even if evil were really only a good, a "residue of experience," as Teilhard de Chardin would say, an effect of growth or an effect of contrast, nothing at all, a lesser good, a good not yet perfect, a detour to lead to an even better good, or a condition for a greater good, there would still be a vague something, an *uneasiness,* which would be sufficient to warrant and to explain why we speak of *evil,* a something we never succeed in entirely doing away with, an "incorrigible." Try as we may, the very effort to overcome our senses in revolt proves what it is trying to ban: the unjustifiability in the reaction of our consciousness and sensibility, in the disharmony, the "incompatibility of disposition," the divorce, "the inequality of myself with my own being," "the insuperable contradiction which is a part of [man's] own being, and which he strengthens by his very act of denouncing that contradiction." [27] Thus, evil rises again from its ashes and appears here as the fire which seemed to be extinguished there. Is the very need of assuming its presence, of overcoming it, of furnishing explanations and antidotes for it, not a supplementary proof of its reality? Believing it to be the accidental instrument of an essential good ("everything is good, and evil originates as an accident of this good") is confirming the presence and the reality of evil, just as refutation establishes the difficulty and repression establishes the riot, with the seriousness of the riot in proportion to the means mobilized to repress it.

Now that we have granted evil an official recognition, we could, of course, attribute it to our will or our sensibility, part of a world not necessarily ordered according to human finality: "Man is not the measure of everything."

Such ways of circumscribing evil are closer to despair than to wisdom, and I see very little to distinguish the absurd world of man in revolt from a world not ordered, as they say, according to human finality. This is where the deep-seated pessimism of certain attenua-

---

uprightness of heart and not the superiority of insight, a frank and sincere avowal of doubt, refusal to make a show of a pretended conviction, especially before God with whom it is stupid to play tricks anyway—such are the only claims which had any effect on Job's divine sentence, such is the advantage of the righteous man over the pious flatterer." (Emmanuel Kant, *Penseés successives sur la théodicée et la religion* [Successive thoughts on theodicy and religion], translated into the French by Paul Festugiére, (Paris, 1931), pp. 151-153, as quoted by M. Nedoncelle, *L'Ancien Testament et les chrétiens* [The Old Testament and Christians], *Rencontres,* no. 36, pp. 76–77).

[27] J. Nabert, *op. cit.,* p. 35.

tions of evil may be perceived. By a paradoxical contrast, a deep-seated confidence in God and a great deal of credit granted to creation and to God, or at least faith in the existence of God, of a perfect God, a God of love, may be perceived in certain exaggerated conceptions of evil which take it *too* seriously. Evil, as I emphasized in the preceding chapter, presupposes, at the least, a universe created for something, for a good corresponding to the requirement for absoluteness inherent in each of us. This desire only has meaning if, implicitly or not, we believe in God. From this standpoint it makes little difference whether or not man is the measure of all things. Even if it is only relative, evil is absolute scandal, a deficiency in the work, by definition and by our judgment.

Evil is only a reality if I believe in God, if I love God and he loves me; otherwise, nothing would have any meaning, and evil would reel right along with the whole world. Now, when we accept that the very notion of evil requires a preceding act of faith in supreme goodness, is it not "a must" that we follow this act of faith as far as its logic leads, until we reach the solution of the enigma it raises?

The unjustifiable suffering of an innocent person: an all-powerful, all-loving God *could not* have wanted it to happen, nor could he have permitted it. My reason refuses to reconcile these two contradictory items of evidence. My reason cannot reconcile my reasons for believing in God and evil: Evil requires both that I situate the world in God and that I abandon that attempt. My reason is confounded, scandalized.

"I don't *see* it," says the believer who has understood the vanity of arguments, "but I hope that there is a solution. I hope so because of my faith itself. *Through it the enigma was born, by it I put myself in God's hands to solve the enigma.* I believe, I hope, that in God the irreconcilable will be reconciled. If I were convinced that there is no possible reconciliation, I would abandon my faith. We can never explain evil, but it is no less true that God has assumed evil, and we do have indications of this: Christ did suffer. We already possess the first fruits, the *earnest* of a certain solution: It is what we call *'hope.'*"

3

Testimony 1: A Heroic-Aesthetic Attitude of Youth

We must not misuse the word *testimony*. I will, however, use it in two ways in this book. The entire last part of this book is devoted to letting testimony unravel the impasse of pain and evil; and at the same time, the very evolution which is indirectly recounted in this book constitutes a testimony, a specific case of revolt and reconciliation. This personal testimony has through the years become evident bit by bit, often separated in time and often without each bit being immediately obvious. In the pages to come, the reader will be able to examine a testimony which reveals my state of mind fifteen years ago. I will not change anything. For me, and I hope for the reader, it is a valid testimony, stages in a whole and in an evolution. It will be seen how I attempted to get out of the impasse: "One can and must, through and beyond revolt, reach optimism, a justification, an exaltation of the Creator God, along that road which so many rebels have ascended, going beyond their own rent souls as attacking men jump the bodies of fallen comrades. . . . A positive solution, a constructive one for the inevitable refusal of evil by our conscience. This refusal does not necessarily lead to crime, destruction, or absurdity. It can lead, if it follows its (heroic) asceticism far enough, to love. . . . Such is the morality which we would like to find, and every morality is found to originate there – if it is true that every one proceeds from a sole and unique desire for *transcendence. Every morality is a form of asceticism. And ascetic effort necessarily reaches the goal, if it pushes far and hard enough, of sacrifice. All moralities, without an exception, even those of pleasure and self-interest, come together in their culmination of love, providing only that they follow their own rules to their logical conclusions.*"

It is already possible to imagine the moral attitude, with aspects of both *heroism* and *aestheticism*,[1] which was leading me toward a solution for the problem of evil both on the level of mankind and of God. "Cosmic evil is not to be explained by human liberty. It can only be justified on the level of divinity, as a liberating act of God toward God himself."

It would be an exaggeration to pretend that I do not recognize myself in this attitude, fifteen years later; we stay ourselves during our personal evolution, whether it is slow or abrupt. Is the error in the coming pages to be found in an excess of logic in the midst of what is beyond logic or in an excess of resentment? Judge for yourself:

> *Evil: A Heroic Act of God (My Statement in 1950)*
>
> As I see it, refusing to attribute evil to God is *either* becoming trapped in a sentimental attitude ("God could not have acted thus") *or else* imprisoning God within attributes with which we have endowed him. Evil, as we have seen, cannot be imputed to a creature: so it must be attributed to the Creator.
>
> Evil, desired by God. A barely expressible mystery: Absoluteness renouncing itself, lifting itself out of itself in order to reduce itself to a relative state, liberating itself enough to put nothingness within itself!
>
> Evil, God's supreme modesty.

[1] For, as we have seen, evil and morality were (and are) united, one dictated by the other (which? I believe that my moral attitude was dictating my vision of evil, which I thought to be dictated by that moral attitude). My formulation was made up especially of challenge and of a love for paradoxes. "Our plan is to show the unity of all sets of morals, *that is,* of all human attitudes in the face of evil. The advocate of individualism is on a par with the advocate of collectivity, the apostle of revolt finally accepts, even conforms to a given morality, *by a trajectory that every one follows to a greater or lesser distance, the end of which is love.* The heroic liberating movement of the individual leads to altruism by an inner necessity which makes every individualistic morality into the anteroom of a dialectic of communication. *The individual is the very organ of that set of values which will disappear when the collectivity appears.* The one who separates himself from God in the most definitive way, says Kierkegaard, is the closest to God. We know that he who loses his life, is saving it.

"The refusal of evil, although it at first appears to shock the spiritual minded person or believer, really comes back and embraces him (in order to smother him?). In fact, to the extent that revolt might succeed in producing optimism, it would merit being called a 'successfully Promethean attitude.' Some will see something worse in it; they may accept some feelings of sympathy at the sight of a Prometheus bound and torn, but what about revolt rising up in the clear air on its own wings? Reaching love by the devilish path of refusal: perhaps unforgivable for the narrowly spiritual minded. Judas himself could have done no better, we hear them cry, nor Satan if he had followed his revolt to the end and then accepted God!" (1950).

Absoluteness making itself other and less than itself: the most elegant humility possible – unless it be that of abandoning this abandonment itself. But abandoning it is the act of consummating it: Abandoning the act of leaving absoluteness is the same as already having left it.

The thought that evil was decided by God fills me with respect for the fearful mystery of evil, augments my respect, my love, and my compassion for God. For in him evil can never be anything but a staggering revolution, a sublime sacrifice, a painful and joyful renouncement.

If there is any *fault,* it is an august *fault,* by which God takes off, like a garment, his marble perfection, his absolute immobility, in order to move the movements of liberty, a liberty in which choice and freedom have come together.

"If, in order to be free, it is necessary to choose between good and evil, God is not free, for he is the one who cannot choose evil," wrote Augustine in an attempt to show that in man "the will, which is free in evil because it finds its pleasure there, is not free in good because it has not been saved." [2] An amusing thought on liberty as far as man is concerned, but its gravity concerning true liberty would convince us if it could be applied to God without begging the question. God, we answer, is free in evil. The proof is that he is free, *and* that he desired evil.

God is not a servant of perfection as a triangle is a servant of its properties. Good and evil spring from his liberty. If he is good, it is because at every moment he so desires to be. And he can stop desiring it, in order to decide evil.

Only God could freely choose evil. Men only commit evil as slaves. God can decide evil, not because of weakness, but by virtue of his strength; not because he might yield to evil, but by triumphing over himself to the point of reaching down to evil.

But can we call evil that which is chosen by liberty, by God? No, *if* we have defined evil as "that which (God's) liberty does not choose." God, at the origin of evil, would therefore not have chosen evil, could not have chosen it by its very definition, since evil only takes the meaning and name of evil on the human level, where it is not liberty but servitude which "chooses" it (if it is possible so to express the very absence of authentic choice). If evil is only that which man's servitude to his own nature leads him to commit, then evil is born, created in and by man. And it

[2] Augustine, *Contra Duas Epistolas Pelagianorum.*

is useless to add that this servitude, even to nature, came from the hands of God, although his free will is only capable of choosing goodness: *Evil is what his will does not decide.* Thus evil only exists because of man who, committing and suffering it, is the only one who stays *on a level* with evil.

Such a relativization of evil to the level of a human "phenomenon," that is, to the level of a particular mental perspective, must not detain us here.[3] My quest is to imagine how evil could have originated, sprung up in God.

God leaves eternity, his perfection. In order to conceive of his own diminution, his own negation, it was necessary to accomplish the miracle of moving out of himself, of no longer being himself, of being both himself and something else (and less than himself), perfect and imperfect. The fullness of "being" backs away and suspends being to make room for nothingness: an exploit which reaches beyond the limits of reason, of which a free God was capable.[4] God was able to decide his own resignation. He stays God and surpasses himself by desiring to be other and less than God — a paradoxical liberating movement which he only could allow himself to accomplish. The idea of evil represents the greatest victory of God over himself (if such words have any meaning on the level of divinity).[5]

Did he desire an enemy who would both do him battle and be himself, a hostile power who was but an emanation of his own power? He desired his eternal creation to be ever in need of redoing, ever to be overcome. His rest is tension ever born anew. Nothing more disharmonious than an infinite God, relaxed like a broken bow, or like a gas which has only gained volume by losing pressure. Who would defend the concept of a *rarefied* God? God is concentration: eternally active against himself.

Is the creation of evil not particularly evocative of an artistic creation? A Heraclitean act, a Sivaite act, above both good and evil. Evil for evil's sake, would say an advocate of art for art's sake.

[3] The reader is referred to the two preceding chapters. Although entirely valid in a phenomenological perspective which includes in evil that meaning in which I am implied (chapter 1), this tautological definition is no longer acceptable in the context of chapter 2 which is devoted to the *explanations* of evil, as we have seen (1962).

[4] The myth of Lucifer is comprehensible only in this perspective.

[5] This whole chapter becomes nonsense if we do not understand it as playing on the two keyboards of divine incommensurability and an anthropomorphological vision of God. Has man ever done otherwise in speaking of God? This is the only excuse for a philosophical Prometheus (my comment in 1962).

Only God could conceive of such an extraordinary thing: evil! From evil, which he was genius enough to imagine, he was wise enough to draw the singular beauties of justice and pardon, expiation and reconciliation. From evil, he was wise enough to draw an inexhaustible source of goodness and love.

Do not deprive God of *his sin*. Sin in God is a manifestation of liberty – although in us it is but a sign of slavery. God *sinned* when he let the universe fall from his lips, a work that was a failure, spread out in space and transitory in time. What could we make of the universe if we did not see in it a sin, a downfall of God into matter, a scattering of God into dust? God renounced himself enough to inflict on himself weight!

He sinned in feeble and sinful man himself: by punishing him, and even more, by redeeming him. The Incarnation was an unexpected derogation committed by God against God. But the weakness he gave himself appears to us stronger than his strength. Redemption is God's absurd weakness, accomplished to enable evil to rise, not to the same level as, but above, good. Such is the inconceivable sin of God which the history of Christianity recounts.[6]

God loved evil. Only he could love it as a result of his liberty without alienating that liberty.

He did infinitely more than to create good with good. Having created evil, having stooped down and raised it up to his level, God produced a *different* good, a *better* good, with evil.

This enemy of good which was not permitted permanently to hold good in check, nor continuously to offend God, this *evil* rejuvenated good. This monster from God's workbench rejuvenated God who, having run the supreme risk in this act, comes back to us with a changed face, unrecognizable, new. His love is different. The evil he did us is no longer an evil.

What happened? No longer do we know what our situation is with him, because of the folly he produced.

We suffer because of him, and he suffers because of us, for us! We expect everything from him, but he is expecting everything of us, and is waiting in *uncertainty*.

Such is the strange situation God made for himself, and for us. Such is the strange sin of God, an act of his sovereign liberty. If sin is the transgression of God's law, then God sins eternally.

[6] May I recall that these pages were written at a time when I was outside revelation—at the door looking in, as it were—and extremely sensitive. This may be seen in the very disrespect they flaunt (my comment in 1962).

—So, you say, what a strange panegyric of evil! Do you not agree, when you get right down to it, that evil ameliorates even good, by a strange mechanism whose secret is kept by God himself?

—Let us make no confusions. Evil is still a scandal. It might not have been. It could have been placed there for our punishment or for our good! But evil does exist: I have tried to understand it in God. If it is no longer possible to justify it in creation, is it not legitimate to explain it as an act of God? Evil acquires a semblance of meaning if we are ready to see in it an act of God moving out of himself (and leaving, if I may say so, his worn-out official uniform). It would almost seem that in evil (and beyond both good and evil) God gives us the example of an act valid in itself, which is wound around its own justification. This act could be the illustration of an ethic.

Or rather is it not by working from an initial moral intuition that I was able to imagine the beauty of the divine act, an act of self-liberation whose worth puts beauty into evil itself? This intuition, which allowed me to understand evil in God, may perhaps furnish us with a *model* of our attitude in the face of evil and pain in this life. Perhaps this intuition of God's act can give us the basis for a moral standard.

This morality is called transcendence.

Evil acquires a valid existence if it is the expression of a heroic *transcendence* of God beyond God himself, an instrument to be used by God, not by us. For evil was not given to man for his good since even *better* was possible for the One who is all-powerful. But we can understand how God, the absolute fullness of good, liberated himself from himself. Now, evil itself is a ridiculous link: Beyond simple good, God could have conceived of a way of *detouring* evil, a complex situation. But even beyond, we find again the simplicity of good. Creation is complicated (even if only in our minds), constantly at battle with itself to conquer itself. But even renouncing transcendence is transcending oneself. Why evil—just to be vanquished? Why sin—just to be destroyed by pardon? A united world, simple, full of grace, must have been possible.

Absolute liberty, gratuitously rich, oscillates between easy and difficult, war and peace, good and evil. Difficulty overcomes itself and finds easiness on the other side of victory, like a greater difficulty. If the weak man's ideal is strength, that of the strong man is to know how to be weak. When it reaches its limit, strength goes beyond itself and becomes weakness. God's strength was able to become weakness. *More* effort is necessary to be weak than to be strong.

But weakness attained by a "show of force" is short-circuiting itself. Any quest is seen to be surpassed by renouncement of that quest: The seeker abstains and rests in peace. God in pain infinitely surpasses all-powerful God, but he is surpassed by other strengths more extraordinary, more distant, more complex – and at the same time, more and more simple, with an immediate yet inaccessible simplicity.

The God of love is but one aspect of that infinite act from which every particular value is derived and takes its substance: the act of transcending self. God is greater in justice, greater in forgiveness or, rather than in either one of them, in that act by which he transcends himself and transcends justice in forgiveness. Would forgiveness have revealed all its worth if it had not been fixed in the setting of necessary justice? In it we see the other side of the punishing God, his gratuitous and gracious decision which fills us with joy. God was able only once to realize the miracle of giving himself to us because he has denied himself throughout eternity. His very denial magnifies the graciousness of the act of giving.

The act of love is victory. God ascends when he descends to the level of his creature, when he holds out his hand to the sinner, becomes himself a creature. God could have spared us all that pain from the very beginning. If we wish to understand the detour of evil, sin, and pardon, we must not think about ourselves but about God: for in him was realized the unheard-of act which reverses all sets of values and puts sinners higher than the righteous – and it is this scandalous act of love which delights us.

The God of love is not "above" the God of justice: but this God of justice transcended him by *becoming,* by *turning around (metanoïa)* in order to be seen in his love. The God of justice decided – an act of ineffable liberty – to cease his justice, to suspend it, to pardon.[7]

But love transcends itself when, overcoming love for the creature, suffering a hundredfold for the suffering it inflicts, it forces on itself the act of punishing without weakness. Overcoming

[7] This contrast between the New and Old Testaments is too schematically stated: God forgave at the Exodus, at the Flood, and even Adam, Eve, and Cain (my comment in 1962).

pardon and overcoming justice are the same thing.[8] The worth of the act does not stop short in either the strictness or the goodness one may reach; but in the lifting motion which carries us from one to the other, in the act of leaving self — of moving out of self in order to change faces, to be liberated from the burden of being what one was!

Among all the moralities proposed by men, there is not one which is not ascetic in nature. This asceticism common to all, which is morality itself, is a result of the antinomies that divide them — for example, the moralities of pride and of humility. *Humility* in the sense of resignation is utterly worthless, and Nietzsche's reaction to it is understandable. But if it is conquered and adopted by an advocate of strictness, it becomes an even greater strictness, one which Nietzsche could have reached had he gone beyond the course he was following.

The divine act by which God decided to permit evil, and to redeem it, reveals to us an ethic: the transitory and dynamic worth of human actions — which are deposed with one act of creative transcendence.

Are justice and pardon complementary like Socrates' pleasure and pain, intimate enough to "hold hands"? [9] I believe in another "theory of opposites": Justice leads to love, not because each is only possible because of the other, but because pardon is obtained by overcoming justice, and justice by overcoming love.[10] God

[8] Nietzsche tried to rise above love in strictness: "Thus speaks any great love; it overcomes even pardon and pity. Woe to those who love without that elevation which lifts them above their pity. God also has his hell: his love for mankind" (Zarathustra). But neither does strictness have anything to make it superior to the supreme weakness of a merciful God. By going beyond the guilt of sin and so reversing the accepted set of values, Nietzsche gains a lap, if one may say, on Christian values, but his lead does not last long for he is, in turn, surpassed by the extraordinary strength of any *obtained* weakness. In 1962 I saw that such a relativistic view of values, no matter how dynamic and exalting it may be, crumbles like a castle in the sand if it is not founded on the will of a God desirous of something for us and associating us with the creation of the world until it is *finished.* This remark, made here only, is valid for this entire chapter—the expression of a theory and a date partially valid and acceptable. *Man in revolt* belongs to every period, and it would be a mistake to underestimate his intelligence and his heart. Are there not illustrious examples even today?

[9] "Although they cannot come together, if the first is followed and attained, the other is almost always taken with the first" *(Phaedo).*

[10] A very closely related idea is to be found in the dialectic of justice and love, each of which exists only if it is the other. There is no justice if it is not inspired by love, no love if it is not justice. From a superficial opposition we progress in depth until we reach the unity of justice and love (my comment in 1962).

lifted us up in spite of ourselves, in spite of himself. It is this *in spite of*, the basic formula for a theory of opposites based on transcending acts, which constitutes the essential point.[11]

"Love your enemies, bless those who curse you. . . ." The exceptional power of these precepts, which sting like so many blows from a whip, is to be found in the desire for the opposite which lifts us out of ourselves and liberates us from our little selves. Injustice brings out anger in us, but soon it is possible for us to answer it with love. Every difficulty is dislodged by grace – as soon as we have found the secret of a liberty which disassembles the mortal chain between indifference and indifference, evil and malice, injury and vengeance. So we manage to leave ourselves and become *other*. What a victory of an attitude over its opposite! This dynamic vision of *opposites* is comparable to Jesus coming after Socrates to bowl over, to turn upside down, to transform values. Happy is the man able to triumph over his own nature and to appear as the opposite of himself, converted into his opposite! That evangelical precept is a whip for us because it exhorts us to be the opposite of what we are.[12]

We may understand, with all this in mind, how a defect can be transformed into a quality by the fact of turning it around. Selfishness and disinterestedness thus lose their officially assigned qualities: Everyone can be selfish or disinterested through disinterestedness, or selfishly he can be one or the other. Disinterestedness sometimes reaches the state of imprudence, folly – and beyond, it reaches that folly of selfishness which only represents a paradoxical superlative of itself: that state of economy and

[11] Quoting Socrates again: "Everything is born of its opposite. Something becomes great because it was small, for it was necessary for it to have been small in order to become great. So it is with good and evil, beauty and ugliness." I would say that something has become great *in spite of* having been small, good *in spite of* having been evil. For it is not only necessary for this thing to have beforehand been small or worse, but (otherwise there is no reason why it did not stay in that state) an effort is also necessary; a creative miracle has to intervene in order to *change* smallness to greatness, evil to good. Each attitude is an obstacle to the one it is denying; as a rival it only asserts itself after transcending its "opposite."

[12] From the same genius are derived the extreme considerations enjoyed by suffering, weakness, and failure in the mystery of Christianity—all so admirably presented in *The Power and the Glory*, by Graham Greene (New York: Viking Press, 1958). Sin, cowardice—these are higher than virtue and strength, as signs of a supreme liberation, signs of power and of glory, *of God;* without doubt, but also they are signs of *the one* who is all by being nothing, who has found all by losing all. The theme of glorious misery is the same as liberty. Supreme liberty is in presenting to God that glory which we have torn from the heart of our own defeat, from our own pain.

tightness due to our accountability to others. Beyond the folly of unselfishness (which can, therefore, reach the folly of selfishness) do we not attain *reasonableness,* that neutral state, so lukewarm that earlier we would have spewed it out? Love was supposed to understand *everything,* forgive *everything,* give *everything,* without measuring or counting; but now it manages to parcel out its goodness, refuses to understand, to forgive, and it forbids itself the "folly of goodness."[13] The price of moderation, of prudence is exorbitant – especially since they have already been surpassed in folly; cowardice and shabby lukewarmness will henceforth be set higher than imprudence, than folly, and will become their very outer limit. It is possible to push imprudence so far as to venture into the dangerous territory of prudence, for the ascetic to risk entering the world of comfort while trying to keep his spirit of poverty. The folly of goodness can only reach perfection by renouncing the summit of folly – moderation, a moderation obtained on the other side of folly. The *same path which surpasses moderation in order to reach folly* surpasses *folly in order to attain moderation.*

Beyond moderation, liberty reaches folly. But, beyond folly itself, it reaches moderation.

The worth of the act rubs off on the movement which makes up the act: whence our tendency to confer on the movement the glory which belongs to the motive behind the act. We may think we admire a hero for the ideal he embodies, but we really love the ideal because it is embodied in that hero.[14] A morality does not make its own heroes, but a hero makes his morality. The

[13] Having taken on himself our errors and having suffered in order that they be redeemed down to the last most unpardonable one, Jesus requires this condition: that the sinner take the first step. He comes near to the one who believes in him and rejects the unbeliever or the Pharisee. But it is the sick who need a physician. This astonishes us at first; then we get used to it. We understand why it is sometimes necessary to force oneself to say no. But how far will this understanding take us? Perhaps it will take us as far as that opportunistic morality which we threw out a moment ago and which is found in some strong advocates of love: "That's the way it has to be, even if I would like to love 'immoderately!' "

[14] Dramatic authors and novelists only succeed in eliciting our admiration for completely opposite actions by bringing them out of a man's self-renouncement. Behind the diversity of dramas, whatever the ideal may be which inspired them, we may discover only one formula, one secret: heroism. This is a truth with fearful consequences, for our admiration will belong to a hero of evil (as is too often seen in novels of war and crime) by the same magnet that draws it to a hero of good. There is a strange conflict between the transcendent motive, which is the essence of the moral act, and the desire for good, which is one of its terms.

greatness of an act inspired by renouncement and transcendence is what gets the movement rolling which bit by bit forms the ideas of justice, honor, and love. These virtues are not illuminating but illuminated: The act is the sun from which they receive light and strength.

"Blessed are the meek." This meekness appears as abandonment, relaxation, but it is tougher than the clenching of fists to which we are accustomed. The joy of this abandonment is the joy of conquest, the joy of war. Peace is a war waging war on itself, a war overcoming itself.[15]

Does this mean that an act is only worthwhile to the extent that it costs us something? No, for merit resides more in the gift than in the effort. But even then, the notion of effort stays on even, and especially, in a transcended, vanquished effort. A merit is all the more brilliant for the small amount of effort and large amount of grace it reveals – provided, however, that we have thought of the effort which would have brought us to that point. The more the effort is forgotten, the more merit there is: but only because the first merit made us think of that act. And it is only by a sort of state beyond effort, where effort is progressively rendered useless, that the absence of effort is appreciated. The greater the effort, the greater the merit; but it is even greater if it was not necessary. *Effort is higher than the absence of effort, and the absence of effort is higher than effort.*[16]

The same impetus runs like a golden thread through philosophies of transcendence and through those of participation, which

[15] Commenting on *Le devoir* [Duty] by Le Senne, L. Lavelle summed up the spirit of the work in these terms: "War must create peace, not a dead peace which is more decisive than war, but an active peace in which separation is ever rediscovered as a means of uniquely voluntary union. We must live in pain in order to struggle toward joy, in bitter duty in order to reach that grace which will make it useless." (L. Lavelle, *Le moi et son destin*) [Self and its destiny]. Lavelle opposes this heroism with "the fundamental experience of participation rather than of contradiction. The world takes us in before it puts us out. What we took for an obstacle was an appeal. Love goes before hate, which itself is nothing but thwarted love." This philosophy of grace is opposed to one of duty; but even that philosophy should have transcended itself to reach peace, beyond the effort of transcendence itself. This "initial" peace, to which it would have been sufficient to open the heart, is a final peace, in that it was necessary to *aspire* to it first, and then to reach it by an effort of deprivation and renouncement. Any philosophy of peace is a philosophy of resolute war.

[16] Charles Péguy wrote, in an entirely different context, "The one who gives up is not giving up and he is the only one not to give himself up. He who does not give up is the only one who gives up. . . ." *Le Mystère des saints innocents;* English translation is *Mystery of the Holy Innocents and Other Poems,* trans., M. P. F. Pakenham (New York: Harper & Row, Publishers, 1957).

are only apparently in opposition, since the first contains the second. I can accept that grace existed from the beginning, but it is grace only if I can measure the distance which separates me from it and the immense liberating flight which it represents for my chained soul. Grace was there, waiting for me: but I had to tear myself away from myself in order to become available and receive it. Peace is a result deserving of itself. Heroism is change, and heroism and peace are only moments of the action.[17] Ease, like difficulty, is a link in the chain which difficulty must follow. The transcendent act, which takes us beyond ourselves, is war and peace, pain and joy, thirst and satisfaction, morality and every set of morals, the very pulse of the spirit.[18]

Human Innocence: From Revolt to Acceptance (My Statement in 1950)

It seemed to me that the mystery of evil could only find a "solution," if a solution were possible, in God and under the banner of a heroic vision of divinity. On this level, evil is no longer constrained to account for itself – it is an act surpassing the perfection of good, an act of God appearing higher than God himself. But on *our* level, evil will never cease provoking painful

[17] Participation and heroism are as opposite as arrival points and points of immobility. They are fragments abandoned in a unique flight of transcendence. Hearing an appeal in the world is no more attractive than seeing an obstacle. Neither is it more attractive to see pain as hindered joy than joy as pain overcome. The only valid movement is the one that lifts us out of both of them. Heroism would seem to have better understood this if, like Nathanael (Gide), it taught us to abandon it in turn.

[18] In the 1950–1952 text a parallel between the "moral act" and the "artistic act" emphasized the aesthetic/heroic quality of the whole movement. This portion would have no place in the present work. But I still feel that "the idea of *beauty* is inseparable from the idea of creation, that is, from a victorious combat over matter, over chaos. The creative artist overcomes nature with an act that reverts to nature. Art triumphs over itself, becomes a slave of nature, as pride gives itself over to the humility of grace. The creative efforts of artist and hero follow the same curve. Like the artistic act, the ethical act transcends nature, then comes back to it and renounces itself in it. The incomparable successes of nature in art and in heroism have no meaning whatsoever if they have no history. We appreciate them to the extent that they have carried an act in history to its culmination. It is in the transcendent act that I understand aesthetic beauty and moral beauty. Both are manifestations of the visible presence of a liberty which has been realized, materialized as it were, in an object or in an act. If the ant or the termite did not reach the total collectivistic gift of self by overcoming, sacrificing individualism, by slowly renouncing its liberty, that gift would be meaningless, and nature is a monstrous absurdity. In art and in morals worth is at the end of a road, of a history, of a transcendence realized in history—and self-effacement is its highest form."

stupefaction, a thirst for justification that nothing can satisfy in any adequate fashion.

What a curious interpretation is that given of the heartrending spectacle of man's goodwill struggling against human nature! We blame ourselves for *committed evil* because of that nature inflicted on us as an infirmity. And the inalienable part which our goodwill contributes (our demand for better), which is *our* part, we try to attribute to God and his grace. Is this not reversing the roles?[19] The impression which crystallizes from this defective humility, full to overflowing with goodwill, is entirely pity and pride. Man desperately struggles in the snares set for him by God. Many are his efforts against the nature he has received, vain and untiring; how deep are his reserves of patience and love! By endowing us with a biopsychology against which our indefatigable desire for the better is constantly breaking its lances, God put us in a position requiring us to judge him – requiring us to forgive him. The hand that God is supposed to be holding out to us, we are untiringly holding out to him. We make all the advances. We make his silence, his indifference to our pain, into merited punishments. We imagine that he is suffering a hundred times what he is making us endure. Man's stubborn love for God: the evil sent to him by God he accepts; he accuses himself of it; and he worships him even more. Nothing can change human acceptance. What is a holy martyr? Someone whom God causes to suffer, who was able to suffer, because of his faith, better than others. How admirable is man's dignity! How right we are in venerating the martyrs!

God gives a high price in pain for what he asks of us. The fact that man's faith manages to partially neutralize this ugliness and pain changes nothing as far as the cruelty and futility of the price of pain is concerned. The principle of pain's usefulness only maintains an ignoble ambiguity. If a mistreated child becomes a stronger adult (God forbid that this be true, and psychoanalysis has shown this pedagogy to be of doubtful quality), we should be happy. Is pain a trial to be borne to make us better? God could have tried man in a way other than pain. Pain only improves strong men, while it grinds down and debases the weak.

[19] Since 1950 I have come to understand, however, that everything I possess, everything I accomplish, everything I give I receive from God. What I wrote then does not appear *wrong* to me; it is true in a certain sense. But in this area, I must add, truth is not separable from our own attitude, our work. Is my present conviction not the end of a curve which I used to foresee as a straight line? (See pp. 174 ff.)

It is not enough in itself; it works as much against man's cause as for it.

One who knows how to endure martyrdom and how to worship the torturing hand is admirable, not the One who permitted the martyrdom.[20] Some want to take the holiness of a few as evidence of divine grace, but this holiness is proof of nothing but a trait of human character. All of God's plagues only provoke adoration in some, but this does not prove that these plagues were good, only the strange goodness of some human characters. We must beware of our simplistic tendency to take for divine love what is only our human love refusing not to believe in that divine love *in spite of everything!* Saying "God is love" is expressing that we are full to overflowing with love for God. Saying "Creation is good" is showing that we are full of goodness.[21] Saying "All is joy and beauty" is giving words to our own joy, which in truth is the greatest beauty in creation.[22]

After all, only our acceptance and love are proper in the face of evil — not because we have recognized any meaning in evil. Any position taken by man which would attribute to evil a hidden good, incomprehensible and mysterious, seems to us to be either hypocrisy or unconscious gullibility, and even worse, a sort of betrayal of God himself. Pretending that God could not have permitted evil (either in the sense that he only wanted it for our good, or that it came into his plan only through our liberty) is *being ashamed of God* and making for him another face because we did not have the courage to accept the one he has.

We must learn how to look evil in the eye, just as it is, without being ashamed of it or of God.

When we have observed the presence of evil, we have the right

[20] The first may be called *holy;* the second cannot be the God we adore. It is better that God not be such; only the absurdity of a universe without God explains the evil which every day causes us to revolt. But that is impossible; from the indifference of nature we must necessarily refer back to the indifference of a God without whom any usage of the terms "good" and "evil" would have no meaning.

[21] The strange goodness we have called to mind here is no less of a problem in its own right, and it is, in turn, an evidence, in one way or another, in favor of a love whose bearer reaches out to us (my comment in 1962) (cf. chapter 4, p. 181).

[22] *Nota bene:* The beauty, in what we might call the active tense, of creation changes nothing in the scandalous nature of evil. In a creation effected by a perfect Creator, good is no problem, only evil. Saying that creation is evil is giving speech to a discontent just as subjective as the contentment which says that it is good. But alone, a subjective discontent is an objective evil, and alone, evil produces scandal and not good.

to refuse it, to combat it, or to ignore it. It is perhaps more dignified to hold out our hand and go out to meet it. The loving attitude is the better, not because evil is good in any way at all, but because it demands that we transcend ourselves. It requires *more* of us, more goodwill, more patience, more renouncement, and more liberty.

Liberty, as it progresses, finally reaches unselfishness, and beyond unselfishness, that selfishness which is love.

In the end, it will be found that creation is good, that evil is a kind of developer or catalyst of good (by it "good" will become "better"); but our human pride goes so far as to assert it now and even to think it is so. If our pride is able to follow its own conclusions to their extreme limit, if it is ready to go to the limit of love, I *will forget* that creation is good thanks to my pride and love. I will end up thinking that it is *inherently* good.

Thus, *by a detour which is in itself all-important,* we come back to the assertion which we earlier termed gullibility: that evil must really be a good, and creation is good in spite of all the appearances. In order to reach this point, an evolution of human unselfishness to its extreme limit is necessary, and even beyond that limit, by a leap that makes its subjective goodness into a universally objective goodness.[23]

This is how we must act: We must neutralize, do away with evil by our acceptance; we must make our immense thirst for love into divine love.[24] And in fact as soon as our love passes like a breath of wind over evil, it vanishes, evaporates, disappears. It really no longer exists! It will be true, therefore; it is true that evil is not and must not exist. This is true because I force myself and manage to understand it, to accept it, and to neutralize it by the acceptance itself. And it is all the truer to the extent that my acceptance *does not know it* and ends up presenting as an

[23] Saying "Creation is good in spite of everything" is therefore either showing oneself to be very cowardly or else very courageous. Nothing looks more like courage than cowardice, nor more like cowardice than courage—or rather courage is the limit of cowardice, its ruin, its cadaver despised and thrown outside the gates.

[24] It is difficult to stop in time without overextending into masochism. There is no sadder sight than that of a man repudiating what he is. However, our renouncement is compatible with the pride of not blushing because of our humanity, even base and feeble, because we know we are transcending it. But it is true that while our humanity transcends and renounces itself, it will forget the very memory of itself, and its *ruin* will seem to be confusable with the cowardly humility of which we were speaking. The laurels of one will be its *finality;* the poverty of the other will be its *initial status!*

objective judgment the fruit of my infinite goodwill, of my stubborn, untiring prejudice of love.

The absurdity of the whole mystery is that it is up to us to choose how the world will appear to us. Our goodwill is entirely responsible for covering evil with dignity or leaving it as is. The meaning of the universe hangs on our decision. Our pride orders us to cover it with the grace of mystery — and evil will only receive this mystery from our grace.

If there is some monstrous pride in thinking honestly that the faith of man is responsible for justifying and taking on itself the evil of creation, for bearing lovingly a fault of God (an extraordinary mission!); if it is a blasphemy to say with a clear conscience that grace and divine love mean that our human love is transcending itself, is projecting itself elsewhere with enough force to escape its initial gravity, *a proffered gift rather than a received gift;* then we will stop thinking that we are stretching our hand out to God and will finally believe that God is the one reaching out to us.

But in this further trial of man's humility, will we not discover a new growth of unselfishness, of love, one more step taken toward a meeting with God; will we not find the same pride we find everywhere else because that is what we are looking for? We are, in fact, looking for pride in the clearest simplicity, whereas it is hidden where it is protected by a thick layer of relished guilt.

Every justification of guilt once seemed to us to be specious; now it seems useless. As soon as the step was taken by others of "integrating" evil as a ridiculous, beneficent, or merited entity, what is to keep us from the next step: *understanding evil itself,* not camouflaging it, but frankly, face to face? Our love no longer needs to justify its lucid blindness by denying or refusing that evil is from God: Its justification is in itself. If it were not, would our love be *love,* a gracious, disinterested gift, in no way a tribute paid to attain some perfection? We must learn how to love evil, not because it is only apparent (it would only be proper then, and not even worth talking about), but because it is really bad. Our love must have the courage to love evil, not only in creation but in God himself. If God permitted the existence of evil, our love, following its transcending movement beyond the understanding of evil in creation, must assume the evil in the Creator. Thus the path followed by our love will be followed to the end, and the stretched-out hand will be stretched out to the end!

The most stupefying aspect of the universe will be the reach and the resistance of man's good will. Tossed from suffering to suffering, man will find the means of claiming all the responsibility for evil and will thus exonerate God. His worship will find a way to love even God's harshness and will love it enough to transform even it into love!

Does man as a last resort accord to God the grace which God denied him?

What a strange relationship there is between liberty and evil! We are so willing to charge the world's evil to the account of liberty (whereas that responsibility rather belongs to the powers of our own nature which threaten us with slavery; if our liberty is responsible for anything, it is good!). But if this liberty does not explain evil, is its mission not, on the other hand, to untiringly oppose it? Liberty alone is capable of assuming responsibility for the evil which does exist, capable of taking it, accepting it, repairing it; in that sense, *it does in fact bear the weight of the evil in creation.*

Liberty, which is not responsible for explaining evil, is nevertheless the only thing that can explain it. This is not because liberty would commit evil, but because it alone would consent to claim that it is the father; not because it would take the responsibility for it, but because it would be ready to bear it! [25]

Original sin is not a proof of our liberty. But *not disputing original sin* is a proof of our liberty!

I have attempted to cross in two directions that abyss which separates man from the strange reality of evil. First, I have described it as a liberating act of God. By this act sin reaches us already justified in a certain sense. Then, coming back by an analogous liberating act, it reaches us "imitated by God" – which raises our faith to the point of loving something that is unjustifiable.

The same intuition which enabled us to understand evil in God himself also obtains for us that attitude which will be ours in the face of the suffering which we must live through; *it furnishes us with a set of moral standards.* But this morality is only

[25] If a *test* for our liberty is provided by choosing good and assuming responsibility for evil, the highest degree of this liberty must consist in embracing and loving evil itself! And if it is true that the being from whom all proceeds desired evil, then liberty is taking the first step toward him, going to him, even understanding him, pardoning him, and loving him. The further he stands from us, the more our faith must endeavor to approach him—*it must assume the whole task!*

derived from the divine act after having been attributed to it. It is because we started with a moral intuition that we are able to understand God, whose act, in turn, becomes a brilliant example of morality. *God reaches evil and, we can assume, responsibility for evil by an act of transcending self* (1950).

I will end here these few fragments of a personal testimony which began on p. 161 which I wanted to present as a *moment* in the philosophical evolution of a mind. I am in a quandary as to how I can express the *nuance* that all this was both right and entirely wrong. My present conviction, which puts no less of the task on man's shoulders than the former, nonetheless belongs to an entirely different world. In fact, the poles have been reversed. For in this problem of evil, man assumes all the work, as we have seen in my prolegomena to evil, yet it is through man's work that evil is embodied and named; it is through the same channel that it loses ground, backs away, and disappears in hope. So I have not changed in this fundamental point. And yet, I have fundamentally changed in the sense that the ultimate source of my initiative – no matter how totally that initiative assumes the task of reaching out to God – is still found in God. All that I can give, I have still received, received from God. So nothing has changed, but everything has been reversed.

4

Testimony 2: Evil—Testimony and Hope

Evil, as we saw in chapter 1, may not be reduced to pure and simple observation; it is both observation and condemnation. That is, it presupposes man's presence, not indifferent, but active and participating, both judge and contestant, but man is also a qualified *witness*. Evil presupposes man's testimony.

Evil, as we showed in chapters 2 and 3, may not be satisfied, if I may use that term, with ingenious explanations. Their effect on us is rather to prove too much; they make revolt even more weighty and serious.

God loves revolt. It bears witness of a more passionate love on the part of men and a more vigorous sense of the living God than the arguments of apology—but this sense of God is either unaware of itself or else it refuses to admit its own existence.

Rather, apologetics and revolt are both questionable in the way they formulate their theses and are, on the other hand, both evidences of a requirement without formulation (that of justification, chapters 2 and 3).

The Apologist and Revolt

Man in revolt is right, a thousand times right, in blaspheming against the God he perceives. He does not want to pass lightly over man's suffering. The innocent one who must suffer is right to incite indignation against that God, and the "atheist" is against such a God, except that by putting on the prosecutor's robe, he unwittingly abandons the cold formal attire of the atheistic rationalist.

Even the "explanations of evil" are evidences of a love and a sense of God's presence which have more worth than the explanations themselves. Doubtlessly by asserting that evil is only a mirage before the eye of mankind, an optical illusion, a sleight of hand, these explanations blunderingly show no respect for the suffering of others, those who refuse the cowardice of facile consolations. In this sense, explanations of evil are undoubtedly insults against the world's suffering, but such was hardly their intention. These philosophers suffer like their fellowmen, and they take care not to forget them. However, they realize that evil is something other than raw suffering, that it includes something else, a judgment passed on the universe, that this judgment can only be weak, partial, and biased.

Evil is a "nothing" sticking to being like a parasite, they say again, another insult against those who suffer. But this explanation was rather meant to be the assertion of another positive reality without which evil itself could not have stood out as such, could not have been qualified and situated as such. Evil exists only because of that other reality which it denies and which in turn denies it. Evil therefore bears witness to that reality of which it is the negation and which is its own negation.

For a thing is only known and only takes on body by the *difference* it shows from another thing. Evil means that we are escaping evil and the world itself by a sort of dimension of ourselves — a nostalgia, a demand, a certain knowledge, and attainment of the perfect good. Evil is part of a greater experience, and it is precisely in comparison with that experience that it stands out by its difference as evil. Thus evil speaks to us of good; it bears testimony for good, for the Spirit, for God and his love — an offended love. But before love can be disappointed, it must exist.

So we discover that the reasons proposed by both sides, although they claim to be opposite, hide "under the table" a unique demand, the same faith. At least we can say that if they are not identical, they are rather close to each other. For there are steps up to the knowledge of God, as there are different levels of faith, from the most profound to the most superficial, from the most secret, unknown even to ourselves, to the most explicit, shining out for every eye to see.

It is just this love to which both the man in revolt and the apologist bear witness, "over their dead bodies," and they are both unaware of their true testimony. The man in revolt does not know that he is doing a favor for God, that he is bearing testimony for him by his legitimate hate and pain, by his just revolt against the One who permitted it. And the apologist often does not know to what extent his dry, sophisticated reasonings reveal, to the eye of one who knows how to read his heart, a real faith, overflowing his soul and involving his whole being in the service of the true God.

The two adversaries prove, not what they were planning on proving, but something else. Both of them are militant advocates – completely unaware – of the same living and secret reality which furnished the unique springboard for both of their arguments and nourished the indignation of one, the zeal of the other.

Behind Explanations: An Attitude

Behind the positions adopted there is indeed a total involvement of the man who adopted them; the positions are only poor manifestations of the deciding force. The reasons given for condemning or declaring innocent these three abstract parties – man, the world, God – have, in fact, a meaning other than reasons, other than "knowledge." They mean much more: They are already action, the faith of total man and his society, a civilization, a history, a world. Human reasons floating in a sea of "knowledge" (arguments for and against) can only touch on an evil emptied of all its substance, an abstract evil which only recalls very vaguely the experience whence it was born.

A "solution for the problem of evil" must not only call on "knowledge," but it must also try to grasp the origin of that knowledge. It must try to make explicit what it implies. It must, as it were, endeavor to psychoanalyze the knowledge itself. Such a solution must take into account what it says, *but also what it does not say,* and what is implied in what it says.

This solution, in short, is not a solution, but a network of references. It involves man both as a total being and the totality of creation. This double reference takes its substance from what we call *tradition,* made explicit in *doctrine.* Tradition is man making his mark on history. And when history is structured into doctrine, it takes in the totality of time and space. It is universal and eschatological.

Every solution for the mystery of evil is dated; it bears the mark of an era, of a tradition to the extent that it sums up the past in the present. Every solution for the mystery of evil is also an anticipation of the future and the meaning of creation; it sums up the totality of history and also blends in with tradition to the extent that this tradition transcends the present and the past and so situates them in a total vision. Tradition differs from traditions.

Every solution has its own accidental particularities and essential implications. Thus, it signifies a conditioning which goes beyond the intellectual options if we are wise enough to discover it. But it also signifies an aim that goes beyond knowledge, and we must learn how to decide what the goal is. Even more important, empirical conditioning in turn betrays the goal which it embodies and partially disfigures it by making it unrecognizable and illegible. In this case also we must be able to discern behind the psychological aspects a spiritual meaning. The first is the path, the sign, the indications leading to the other; and the second provides the meaning of the first. Let us study this point in a bit more detail.

Ignorance Aimed at God

We said that a concrete "solution" for the "problem" of evil must necessarily be based on something besides "knowledge." On the order of "knowledge," a solution can only be ignorance – but an ignorance pointed toward a reality which is thus shown up and indicated by that knowledge/ignorance.

How can we reconcile evil and a perfect God? And God *is* necessarily implied if evil exists. Our reason is helpless to understand it. Such contradictions disconcert us; evil requires that God be love and without love, all-powerful and powerless, perfect and non-perfect.

But if knowledge here may be confused with complete ignorance as to what really goes on inside, if it can never tell us how God and evil manage to work out their problems together (just as it can never say who God is) ; on the other hand, this ignorance does appear to have received an orientation, to have been turned toward a pole, and this with a remarkable and undeniable obstinacy which is all its own and which we must now endeavor to elucidate.

We know nothing about all this, but we do see in what direction we must turn our ears, our eyes, and our necks.[1] We just may make some progress in that direction if we understand clearly that it is only an opening to a beginning which is very limited and very obscure. We suffer, and God loves us. But God is only accessible to us by his relationship with his creatures and in the language and historical mentality of the latter. He is completely inaccessible in his nature – or only to the extent that he reveals himself, which is insignificant. The notions backing our statements concerning God are vaguely analogical, rather negative than positive, and indicative more than anything else of our attitude as believers,[2] of an "intentionality based on faith." The medium that we have to de-

[1] According to an expression used by the Apostle Paul.

[2] This is all we were saying in chapter 3 but in another way and with a different emphasis—which enables us to say that God's love for us is only an image of our thirst for love.

scribe the object of our faith is the reciprocal description of the covenant — and then not as a detailed plan or outline, not the content, but a glimpse only, just a form. This form clearly designates the object we were seeking, its correlative reality — and it leads us there with all the surety of a high-power drill going through soft wood, of a guided missile streaking toward its target.[3]

Such considerations, known by everyone, enable us to "thaw out" some of the meticulous explanations of evil which we find in such great numbers. All that is necessary is to put them back into the current of ignorant and believing intentionality where their origin is to be found (lest they forget that origin), into that movement which is both questioning and readiness, acceptation and waiting (or hope).

Yes, we must upset those dogmas and "explanations" whose wide-eyed confidence both reveals and betrays true faith. They would lead us to believe that they "have the answer," whereas we have barely begun our search. Faith is not knowledge; it is a journey, a life, an act. It does not have its object in possession (just as truth may not be *possessed*) because it does not belong to the category of having but of *planning,* which is a first approximation of hope.

Possessing an explanation and the certainty of observation, as we saw above, are forms of ignorance which consider themselves to be knowledge, ignorance unaware of itself. With evil, as with everything that concerns the meaning of creation, our knowledge is not possession but project, a kind of "bursting toward" (according to Sartre's excellent formula). The movement which carries us to the borders of evil[4] is a centrifugal movement of transformation, of *requirement,* not a centripetal movement of gathering information *(observation).*

Now, this "bursting toward," which points its fingers, as it were, toward the object without distinguishing its details, *this bursting is love.* Whether its emphasis is that of apologetics or of revolt, of honey or of gall, the anxious look turned toward heaven is inspired by love, that is, a demand for goodness, for perfection, for happiness. This demand includes whatever content each person gives it,

[3] We have tried to show elsewhere to what extent religious psychology (and atheism, which is only one aspect of the latter) shows the reality of its object: God. The logic is analogous here. For it is not a question of providing proof for the reality of God (the notion and term "evil" were enough for that, as we have already emphasized), but of showing how our love for God is a sign of God's love, that evil (which is inseparably our attitude in the face of evil) is an incomprehensible sign of that love which flows in a double current, a love in which our part is not discernible from God's.

[4] "Evil" here is a shorter way of saying the "problem" or the "mystery" of evil.

whatever countenance: love as a goal, love as a demand, or love as a *form.*

This love as a *form,* pure demand and pure tension, a goal, a bursting toward, proves the objective value of love, just as religious psychology with its metamorphoses proves the reality of God.[5] This love is a missile-head with an internal guidance system like those in today's giant missiles. And the head is directed, not by the launching pad but by the target.

In a similar manner, Kierkegaard showed that the object in question is implied by the sight itself: "An infinite desire is desiring the infinite. An infinite worry is worrying about infinity. . . . Whatever the direction may be, the speed of the arrow makes the target jump with the violence of its impact." [6]

In the midst of a dialectic which so closely associates the demand for and the reality of its object — man's loving flight and the object, the source of love in God — it is an abstraction to distinguish between the terms of the exchange within the exchange itself. It is senseless to distinguish the burst toward God — with suffering and evil as its by-products — from God's movement toward his creature; the love we have for God from his love for us. It is certain that we know his love for us through our love for him, but ours is the sign of his. Our love for God and his love for us make up a sole reality of which we can perceive one of the facets, like the back and the front of a single object. This unique reality may therefore be *expressed* in two different and partially opposed ways. The believer will say that our love is received, like a satellite illuminated by the sun, that our love has its source in God. The unbeliever will see in this love, which we consider God's, only an extension of our human love imperiously projected into infinite obscurity and silence.[7] Both expressions also provide strong evidence that our "knowledge" of God and of evil is concentrated into the narrow, pointed arrow of our aim. This aim is love; this loving aim is already in itself an aspect of God's reality because of the dialectic which connects the aim with its object. But the divine reality defined by the term "love" is still *form,* not content. Like the knowledge which expresses it, this love is purely formal. It designates

[5] Compare note 3. This idea should be compared with the Cartesian proof taken from our idea of perfection; if perfection cannot come from us, imperfect beings, it necessarily comes, therefore, from a perfect Being whose reality is thus proved.

[6] In J. Wahl, *Etudes kierkegaardiennes* [Kierkegaardian Studies] (Urin), p. 277.

[7] See chapter 3. The terms used there will perhaps be better understood now.

God, as it designates our knowledge of God, by the purely formal point of an aim, a demand.

But this demand, this aim, is knowledge and more than knowledge: It is action, a testimony in which the entire person is involved.

Action Against Evil, a Seed of Truth

I have purposely used above this word "knowledge" because the term is so disparaged in today's world and in order to restore to it that existential fullness which includes unformulated intuition, experience in life, personal history, "subjective" testimony, and practical action. Abstract knowledge soon reaches the rectangular limits of its little pool where the water is clear and shallow. Beyond, the waves become dark and threatening, and the wader soon finds the water going over his head. There the philosopher no longer reasons; he acts; or else he tells a story, a parable. His language leaves rational ground and takes refuge in paradox and symbol. Knowledge loses its reputation of purity and neutrality. In spite of its flat superficiality, rational knowledge expresses without words, unawares, a deep personal, social, and cosmic existence; the most unimportant syllogism presents to us the visible side of an invisible history and innocently sums it up before our eyes. Our epoch has given itself the task of restoring this depth of history and has been able to make depth understood.

Behind the knowledge which we formulate, there is an unformulated, implicit knowledge which nevertheless finds itself formulated in our words and must therefore be discovered behind the obvious. There is a "knowledge" of the body,[8] a knowledge which our actions and manner of life betray and to which they bear witness. The Marxist term "praxis" has rehabilitated this knowledge which is inseparable from action and sometimes exclusively action, behavior, the experience of living. Thus we are brought back to an old human tradition, the best example of which is found in the Bible: Knowledge is both action and a personal history which is told. Knowledge is not to be found so much in general formulae as in a personal anecdote.[9]

[8] Cf. Jacques Sarano, *Essai sur la signification du corps* (Neuchâtel: Delachaux et Niestlé, 1963). English edition is *The Meaning of the Body* (Philadelphia: The Westminster Press, 1966).

[9] It is significant to hear a great Marxist philosopher tell his own story in his philosophy. "I can already hear the reader exclaiming: 'Dear sir, dear philosopher, you are not serious. You recount your life, your little stories, and claim, moreover, that these solutions are valid on a cosmic scale. What a joke!'" H. Lafebre, *La somme et le reste* [The sum and the remnant] (Paris: la Nef, 1959), p. 11.

As we have already said, objective knowledge necessarily presupposes, whether we agree or not, an adopted position, an attitude of cooperation or noncooperation with the world. *In turn,* cooperative action constitutes a genuine knowledge which does not yield an inch — in fact, the opposite is true — to verbal or general knowledge. We have learned to ask the opinion of the man who "has nothing to say," who does not know how to express himself, or who likes to keep quiet. We press him for his opinion because we are certain that he has "something to say," because he has lived in such and such a condition, because he has put his hand to the plow, has worked, has put much exertion into such and such an area, because he has acquired long experience — the farmer in his earth, the mechanic in his dirt and grease, the militant organizer in his factories, the missionary out in the brush, the physician with his patients. Today the one who speaks too well about anything is easily scorned, and the one who does not know how to speak but how to live, whose life is a compendium of irreplaceable knowledge, is questioned avidly. And he does not know how to express his knowledge! We are the ones who must translate his words.

Thus it is with the man who has suffered in life because of others and for others, who is educated by suffering. He refuses to allow himself to judge, does not deviate from his own line of conduct, continues struggling against discouragement and suffering itself, *in order to bring about change.* He does not accuse; he works for something better. He feels obscurely or lucidly that he is responsible for the very task which will bring about the destruction of evil; he cooperates in the work of diminishing evil. His part is modest, but he does give that much.

What does this man of cooperative action, this man of testimony, have to teach us? I can see him now, harassed by the television newsmen, microphones held out to his word-sparing lips, the star of all the evening news reports! His unshakingly effective devotion gives him the right to knowledge, not of words, but genuine knowledge, which we must try to restore in clumsy phrases, as we would try to reconstitute the journey of a heroic interplanetary explorer. The man who knows what suffering is "has the right to speak." If his purpose is not to condemn but to cooperate, he has the right to be heard; "he has his reasons" for saying what he says.[10]

We must not, for any reason, scorn or neglect such an experience

[10] We must, nonetheless, psychoanalyze his reasons in turn. An attitude is true, not because of the reasons provided for it, nor even by the motivations hidden within it, but by its aim, its meaning.

in the study which now concerns us, nor must we reject it on the pretext that it is illogical and incoherent. It *does* in several ways appear illogical, since it is concrete and expressed in paradoxes and contradictions. It constitutes a living knowledge of evil in which evil finds itself destroyed, that is, adopted, transcended, utilized. It is a knowledge which is action and so anticipates the solution itself, which finds that solution because it invented it, because it is unstintingly bringing it about.

Does such an experience of suffering lack *objectivity*? Of course. No one can escape that lack; the man who claims logic refuses to cooperate with what he calls an *observed* evil, shows himself to be just as "unobjective" as the man who obstinately insists on cooperating, on hoping. The man of noncooperative "observation" is just as unobjective as the man who cooperates but who demands progress. Objectivity here means noncooperation. Such is its true name, and such is its true nature as an attitude of complete man in the world, here an attitude of refusal.

The line of division does not fall between objectivity and lack of objectivity but between two concrete attitudes. They are to be separated according to the criterion of effectiveness, or, which is the same thing, by the criterion of a more or less total comprehension of reality.

The word "objectivity" designates an "objective attitude" which because it is an attitude, destroys the very objectivity which it claims as its own, goes beyond and deeper than objectivity and so reaches the truth of man and his greater or smaller capacity to comprehend and accept reality.

This is the point where effectiveness and truth converge. The attitude of noncooperation is a knowledge which *brings about,* as it were, what it claims to have observed. It is an order of reality in which *observing* is *deciding;* it gives body, consistency, existence. One who claims to study the problem of evil and to *observe* the lack of any justification, of any acceptable solution, does, in fact, not find any solution, *because of his own attitude.* Noncooperation (or despair) realizes at the same time both its effectiveness and its ineffectiveness, its truth and its error: I am referring to its negative effectiveness and truth—inseparable from each other. The impasse is only observed because someone has actively contributed to it.[11]

[11] This is why Cassandras are so ambiguous. They are accused, and doubtlessly the accusation is false, of producing the woes which they only prophesied. But their clearsightedness does take on the significance of an active contribution to the event—an assertion which would undoubtedly be considered false by a rational mind. But what would you think of a doctor who repeated to his

What is the opposite attitude, that of cooperation? An active knowledge, action-knowledge (praxis) first shows itself as an attitude, an adopted position, living partiality. As such an attitude shows itself clearly to be partial, it destroys its partiality. Realizing that it is implied in the very question of a problem of evil, this realization is a psychoanalysis which engenders truth. Cooperation is a knowledge originating in its action, by a kind of bounce-back effect. While it acts in favor of creation, against evil, the effectiveness of cooperation produces a real solution which surges back as knowledge and hope. By *effecting* a solution for the difficulty (called "evil"), it secretes a knowledge; it builds a truth. By so acting, it causes it to be so.

Cooperation experimentally procures energy and joy. Its effectiveness, so proved by the equilibrium and intensity of its life, the good that it produces in itself and around it, is the seed of a truth (proof provided by the fact, the *fait accompli)* in the sense that *by cooperation* a door is unlatched which opens onto a solution of the problem. Evil is seen to be at least partially disarmed, converted. It has changed its name, has taken on a new meaning; the scandal is no more; the difficulty is resolved; the impasse opens up, the knot undone. Thus effectiveness produces truth; it furnishes proof by the accomplished fact acting against verbal arguments.[12]

Men of argument always reply that this effectiveness, and hence this truth, are minute, that suffering never exhausts itself, that it wells up everywhere like water in holes dug in the beach. You may be doing away with the reality of evil — but on such a small scale!

The cooperative attitude does not deny such a statement, but affirms it.

The cooperative attitude does not deny such a statement. Truth for this attitude does not exist apart from the attitude. Truth is established by that attitude. Truth always exists more or less in terms of our complicity. Evil is true. It is less true if we struggle against it; it will not be more if we manage to interject our truth — a truth yet minute, but undeniable and valid if we accept that

patient, "You're lost; there's no hope"? You would think that he was contributing something to the situation. Saying is never ineffectual. And so we involuntarily add a reason to accept as a crime any word or action that is "harmful to the morale of the nation (or the army)." We must also ensure that this "morale" is justified by the cause it is defending.

[12] There are doubtlessly joyous ignorances, "religions for the people," a simple workingman's faith, but the absence of justification covers a fragility which must have its mask of apparent effectiveness removed. Such a discriminating diagnostic is hard to realize in truth, but great trials bring about the division, as do God's judgments which are beyond our fathom.

the world is only beginning. Truth is not only the present, but the future, also. Do the words "human nature" define who I am, or do they rather designate the calling which I sense within myself and do my best to carry out? So it is with the truth of which we are speaking. Is it what our discouragement claims to *observe* — and which is in a certain sense true, with a dead, static, abstract truth? Or is it not also, and much more importantly, what is coming about, what is reaching out and becoming truth? Truth belongs to the future; that is why it is to be identified with the slightest grain of cooperative effectiveness. We may deny that an acorn is an oak, but to say that is probably truer than to say that an acorn is only an acorn: The oak is its total truth.

To the extent that my initiative accomplishes a transformation in the world, it is producing *truth.* Evil may not be reduced to a static problem; my experience interrupts its data, but my work, my vocation, and my testimony do also. These factors must be taken into account by anyone who attempts an inventory of these data. The solution is dependent on them; it is a living solution, constantly changing. The alteration of any part, as in any organized structure, requires a rearrangement of the rest. The reality and truth of evil depend on me, change with me. This truth, which is the raw data for our knowledge, becomes something different through my very cooperation. Therefore my cooperation *is* truth, *is* knowledge, in the sense that it establishes them; they emerge from the reality *which I created.* We are dealing with what one might call an operative truth, an operational knowledge. And this operational knowledge teaches me a knowledge expressible in words; it is called hope.

Cooperation, Source of Understanding

As we have just said, the two forms of knowledge, cooperative and noncooperative, are differentiated, not according to the standard of objectivity, but according to that of effectiveness. Objectivity is sleight of hand: *Fortunately for this objectivity,* noncooperation is no more objective than its opposite. As an observation meant to be objective, fortunately it also bears witness to the complete man, to a truth, and it reaches a depth, an entire area of which it had no inkling itself. There is a richness, a third dimension, at the bottom of this so-called "objective" truth which gives to it a meaning which goes beyond its own. The division is therefore to be made not according to objectivity, which is like an ephemeral skin of truth, but according to effectiveness.

Acting against evil is transforming the data of the problem of evil. This effectiveness is of such a nature that it engenders truth, which we may in turn call "operative" in order to emphasize its embodiment at the heart of our very action. By my action I intervene in the mystery of this world's meaning.

Now, speaking of the meaning of this world, as long as I am cooperating in its realization, is the same as saying that I *understand* it. Cooperation, on the one hand, and capacity for total understanding, on the other, form two facets of man's unique position in the world. We have spoken of one as operational knowledge. Let us endeavor to explain the other as a kind of total knowledge, eschatological. The first is a *witness;* the second is *hope;* and both are one and the same passion in man, that of love.

Bearing witness is (confers) a particular knowledge which we must then understand in terms of hope, that is, in terms of *totality,* of *anticipation.*

Noncooperative knowledge is satisfied with *observing:* It cuts itself off from the current of creation; it becomes sterile; it dries up both the fountain of effectiveness and the fountain of truth *(fortunately,* it bears inescapable proof in another way, as we have seen). It neglects to take into account a great many of the elements in the debate. For observing is abstractly extracting some elements and not taking into account the *entire* experience.[13] Thus the

[13] J. LaCroix, in a study on work which appeared in the *Cahiers de l'Institut de science économique appliquée,* I.S.E.A. (March, 1963), series M, on 16, pp. 16–17, expresses perfectly the revolution which has invaded the very heart of scientific thought: "This characteristic of thought has become obvious in modern science which itself has been transformed from contemplative to operative. In older classical physics, the scientist always stayed at a certain distance from the world he was studying. Every phenomenon could and had to be integrated into eternal laws formulated quantitatively. Measurements could not modify the things being measured. There was no knowledge without reserve and disengagement; it was the notion of observing that predominated. The world was a problem, an object set before the subject who acquired knowledge. Today, knowledge is no longer considered as a spectacle but as work. Modern philosophy emphasizes that man is a being-in-the-world, that he maintains with nature a reciprocal relationship, a dialectic, that there is an indissoluble relationship between the observer and the observed system. Adopting an expression used by Eric Weil, modern physics is *interventionist.* The world ceased being a representation when man became desire: a desire for power, for administration, and, as Bachelard has said, for polemics. Thus Bachelard's epistemology does not consist of description. Only what is seen may be described. And seeing implies inaction; it evokes a dangerous contemplation of ideas. Over against this logic of theories we may henceforth find an epistemology of approximation which demonstrates the solidarity of theory and application, of idea and realization. The concept has become operative. Technique correlatively applies an algebraic formula. Militant rationalism is not a contemplative form of thought, but constructive. Even in mathematics it is thought put to work."

classic scientific method proceeds by isolation from several data. In order to simplify things we can say that noncooperative knowledge realizes elementary experiences — a reflex, for example — then it believes itself capable of concluding that it has in its possession an elementary element of reality. But these experiences are not experience itself. Real experience is identical with hope. What does noncooperative observation neglect?

To begin, it neglects the fact which we have already emphasized, that my cooperative testimony is one datum entering into the problem and contributes to the total truth of the world concerning which we at first only possess some data. These data exist through us, and some are yet in the future.

In the second place, we must accept that the world is not yet finished, and we can say nothing about it before its completion at the end of time: Knowledge itself is eschatological. In the clearest of terms, such knowledge has the name "hope." Hope provides a foundation for that daring anticipation of the future and the end of time. Based on revelation, justified by the assurance given to us by God himself in the covenant and in his Son, hope is a tremendous knowledge which one could neglect only through carelessness when faced with a problem as great as the problem of evil.

For those who would yet repeat that hope comports no knowledge worthy of the name, that it may be reduced to a movement of "animal-like minds," to a pure movement of affectivity, of fear, of mythical consciousness, we can only refer to our preceding considerations, particularly to chapter 1 of Part II. There we studied the importance of what was implied in any so-called *objective* knowledge, scientific, rational, or philosophical. The truths of observation do not exhaust the entirety of truth. Finally, no truth ever concerns an object without concerning the subject it observes; it is a mixture of subject and object. I would like to come back to this point to show how hope encroaches on evil.

Evil: Inseparably a Category of Mankind and of the Universe

Evil is inseparably a category of mankind (by this I mean that it is a category of human revolt in its action and its judgment of the world) and a category of the universe.[14] Thus, evil has both a subjective *and* objective reality, a weight of reality which no dialectic could explain away as an illusion or an appearance. In this sense it is true, but not altogether true, to say that without man the

[14] Cf. Part II, chapter 1, pp. 125 ff.

world would be *neutral* (neither good nor bad), for without man the world is inconceivable, just as much so as a squared circle. The very definition of the world includes the subject by which a world may be defined. I am the one through whom the world is a world, but, nevertheless, I am a by-product of the world: inseparably a subject and an object of the world, eternal and temporal.

The world exists therefore in terms of man; it is a world for man — or else it is not. And evil is only that "lack," that "incompleteness," that division deep within man and his world. Evil is the immaturity or the lack of maturation of the world, to which man gives the name "evil," the meaning of evil, because he "suffers it" as evil. Suffering thus, man acts as the herald, the spokesman of the cosmos. He qualifies both *what is* and *what causes it to be.* He causes it to be even if it is only by his act of qualifying it. Evil is the language of being, and man is its privileged interpreter.

We must come back to evil and pain seen as the language of being, but now we must emphasize this veritable compromise of man in the evil which he is apparently only observing and suffering.

An integral part of the cosmos, man is also its interpreter, and his language contributes to the appearance of evil because by language the very notion of evil is constituted. But man also contributes to evil by his action which goes against the current of the world's growth, by his destructive opposition, his passivity, his revolt, and his pride. His is a double contribution to evil, in reality only one (if we go to the bottom of things) with two different aspects. *The human logos is both an expression of the world and opposition to the world.* It could not be one without being the other, without compromising itself by adopting the garb of the other. Expression is opposition because it is self-asserting; it is enough for it to be one in order to be the other. Evil signifies both of these aspects and our understanding of the term unites them admirably. *Our condition is inseparably the expression of the world and opposition to the world.* The dualism of opposition (or of self-assertion) characterizes us just as well as the monism of expression, and it is impossible for either the advocates of dualism (we are two in the world) or of monism (we are the expression of the world) to claim to be exclusively right.

Yes, the fact that humanity exists is involved in evil by the double mechanism of language (the judgment of the world) and of liberty (opposition to the world). But even this double mechanism speaks in the only language which could not express the world without a certain opposition to the world. It is impossible to pass judgment without a stopping of the action which permits the judge to see every detail of one frame but also perturbs the projection of action. This halt (in the double meaning of the term – both stopping and arresting) is almost a police action: a brutal halt, an aggression. Expressing is objectively fixing. It is naming, and giving a name is having an advantage over reality according to ancient biblical tradition.

With this in mind, we must affirm both that evil constitutes a material reality, that it is an integral part of the cosmos, and that nonetheless man causes evil to exist. The abstract assertion that without man the world is neutral (without the sense of either good or evil) could be true if it were capable of meaning. If the world without man is an empty word, then it would be proper to reintegrate evil into its place (do we dare call it objective?) in the materiality of the world; it would be proper for the world of which evil is an organic part to take responsibility for it. It would be totally improper for the world to ignore evil. The world must accept its responsibility for pain both as a fact and for what it means.

Evil is in the world, a world of which man in turn is an integral part. He also is interdependent with the world. It would be the same thing to say that *evil is of this world* and that *evil is of mankind;* it is twice over of this world, because of the human race.

It would also be the same thing to speak of *evil suffered* by man (suffering, pain) and of *committed evil* (sin), of metaphysical evil and moral evil. I know that here I am locking horns with a fundamental distinction, considered as a precious conquest of the human conscience over the original lack of differentiation which mixed suffering and sin. That conquest was in fact progress, a decisive acquisition of mankind. When this differentiation was made, suffering could no longer be chalked up to sin. This was an enormous deliverance, for Job's suffering grew with every reproach from his friends, reproaches which were in fact the justification of his sufferings. Guilt redoubles suffering. The suffering of an innocent child forces us to find someone else who is guilty. This justification by reference to sin was doubtlessly meant to appease the revolt incited by suffering, but on the contrary it exasperated it. It is doubtlessly true that the desacralization, the demystification which looses suffered evil from the indifferentiated mass called "evil suffered because committed," comes as a liberation of man. Henceforth, he can frankly stand up to the blow. No longer does he need a camouflage which is only an insult to his manhood. Now he can accept the hard reality of the facts. We must not make any confusion in the categories with which we are dealing; we must sow no discord in our own thought. Yes, we do sin, and these sins do bring on suffering; that we must accept. But there are forms of suffering which no sin can justify, as when an innocent child is struck, even if the law of human solidarity is in force. Our modern conscience can no longer accept this sort of barbaric justice which brings the sins of the fathers down on the heads of the children to the thousandth generation. Original sin is no longer accepted in that way – if it ever was.

We carefully separate suffered evil and committed evil, and other languages express these two categories by two different terms. However, if we can designate both of them by the term "evil," this very designation can furnish us with a lesson. If we cannot *go back* to the primitive undifferentiated state from which we happily escaped, we can find a lesson leading us to reflect on this condition indissolubly ours which I mentioned above: both dualistic and monistic. We must understand the broad sense of participation and complicity in which suffered evil and committed evil are intimately confused. Man is both expression and reaction, and expression itself constitutes a reaction. Taken as a whole, man expresses and contributes; he contributes by expressing; and no one knows the measure of each. Therefore, it appears impossible to me to separate (although we may always distinguish) evil caused by man from that evil of which man becomes conscious.

It is two different things to cling to the initial undifferentiated state and to go beyond the differentiations we have acquired without denying them. The problem of liberty and sin intervenes mysteriously but surely into the problem of evil considered as a whole. This intervention, a thousand times over asserted by mythology, seems to me to be due to existential categories rather than to those of rationalism. It is impossible to argue or to contest the fact of this intervention; it can only be discerned, plucked out of the air by a kind of flair, a partiality, a passion, and a faith of which the rationalist correctly would be wary. Considering the position occupied by suffering, it is without the shadow of a doubt impossible to confuse suffering with sin and even less to attribute it to sin. On the contrary, the evil we commit refers us back to the entirety of evil suffered by the entirety of the world (see chapters 2 and 3).

So evil is found in that world of which man is an intimate part.

And man *contributes* to that evil, both by expressing it and by adding to it, if we may say so.

Evil, a category of human revolt to the extent that revolt is a sign of evil, constitutes a part of the world itself, and the meaning of evil is thus included in the meaning of the world. This meaning is a part of the world, but is nonetheless a "second" entity beside the world because it expresses a part of the world: the fact of pain.

Evil belongs to the world, is a moment of the world, a wound in being itself, in reality itself — a nothingness in being, a fault in being. *Evil as a human category is nevertheless an expression of evil as a reality in the world.* Both. And we do not see how one could be anything but the other: We have only found two ways of saying the same thing.

The Identity of Experience and Hope

But, someone replies, does the scandal then not reappear? I have just accepted that evil does not exist *only* because of man and through man. Why then does it cause all of creation to groan? From there we fall back into the habitual "explanations," such as original sin, which I showed to be characterized by abstraction (they are in fact concrete because of that to which they unwittingly bear witness "behind the scenes" of their own formulation). Those explanations are abstract which put the burden of evil onto man, the world, or God; an indissoluble solidarity links evil with man, the world, and God, and man plays his mysterious part in that bond even if it is only due to his position as spokesman for the world — the one who gives it meaning. Consequently, if the problem reappears in the unexplainable presence of universal evil, it is in another fashion: no longer *there before* man who must judge from "out of the picture," but in a union of solidarity with man who has compromised himself by his knowledge (and) his act of opposition (both, but they are one). Man is immersed in his situation; no longer can he relieve himself of the responsibility for evil from which he tried to separate himself by accusing the world, by "washing his hands" of it all.

He must, therefore, take things as they are; he must take his position. He must assume his double role of creature and creator (or as someone has said, as "co-creator") of the world in childbirth. He is co-responsible, both because he is a microcosm of the world and because he is of the world. From this standpoint, it would be ridiculous to *accuse* the world of one thing or another, of being this or that. We must work from the fact as it exists and endeavor to find a meaning for it in the totality we comprise. Thus evil will acquire a meaning, but it will not be initial. It will be *final,* in terms of what we do with it and what God does with it. What the world becomes will retrospectively give meaning to evil; *it will have meaning.* Evil has eschatological meaning: The end gives meaning to the beginning; the future must be included in the present, must precede it, as it were, in order that we might *understand.*

And the language we use when the future precedes the present is that of *hope.* A study of evil must necessarily lead to a *theology of hope.*

If we desired to speak of a language of hope, the translation into words of this living praxis would break that praxis up into notions which one must be content with listing as nomenclature. But hope is life which transcends and unifies them with one bounding movement.

Hope is, first of all, a knowledge of our entire history. It is prophetic knowledge, knowledge by anticipation. Many have correctly refused to reduce the prophet to the ridiculous role of predicting the future; let us leave these games to the diviners with their oracles and soothsaying. However, although prediction is in itself nothing, it does represent what we might call the small change of a total vision, of a real comprehension of God's plan. The prophet is able to *listen;* and, as a very secondary corollary of this, he is able to announce what will come about. The people, of course, feel drawn especially by prediction, just as the crowd in Jesus' time paid attention only to miraculous healings. Both prediction and healing are worth no more than the change handed out by a rich man passing through a crowd of paupers.

The prophet listens; he *waits.* But his waiting is a prayer, a supplication, perseverance, an appeal, a combat — best symbolized in the vision of Jacob struggling with the angel. It would be false to think of a passive, submissive examination. We might better say that hope is a mysterious alloy of the most absolute submission with the most insistent questioning. The prophet "picks a fight" with God; he seems even to be trying to force an explanation from him; he burdens him with troublesome questions; he is not afraid to be the devil's advocate; he dares to speak to this Father whom he adores and tell him that he does not agree. He dares to ask: "How is it that the unrighteous man lives in prosperity and the righteous man is destroyed?"

The strange sound of quarrel and revolt is enough to bring a triumphant smile to the lips of any rationalist, but yet significant of the son's best obedience. Who, besides the one who misunderstands God, or who on the contrary knows him most intimately as one knows one's own father, would so quarrel with God? Between these two extremes we have another set of *scruples:* We are reserved, like good, well brought up little children; we call our respectful distance "the sense of divine transcendence"; we are careful not to be too bold in our demands, neither must we ask too much in homage and adoration.[15] The rough language of a son, the intimate language of the covenant, the passionate, demanding, jealous sound of shared love – such is the prophet's language, such is the language of hope. The jealous believer speaks to the jealous God without observing the conventional forms of politeness, in a truth that nothing sweetens or makes bland.

What is there that gives the believer this assurance in the very heart of insecurity, of fear, faced with the most disconcerting evil? It comes from the fact that hope is a certainty that goes beyond all scientific certainties (which are not much more than probabilities). *We usually set belief over against knowledge.* I "believe" when I do not "know," when knowledge is beyond my reach. If I were able to know, I would not need to believe. But the two terms should simply be reversed. When I claim to know, all I am doing is supposing, setting up certain possibilities, or calculating such and such a coefficient of indetermination or uncertainty. When I say I believe – *if, however, I do truly believe* – I lay claim to absolute knowledge, because it is of another order, of an order in which probabilities are destroyed, as are all the forms of relativity. Here we are not speaking of a patient progression through prudence, methodical doubt, and reason to a set of conclusions which are ever to be doubted anew. We are dealing with revelation, the word of God himself. When someone tells me something, I credit his words according to who he is. When this someone is God, I therefore credit his words according to his stature (this is *petitio principii,* of course, but I am not trying to argue here, but to get something across; I am not demonstrating, but showing, trying to *open eyes).*

Yes, hope is simply crediting God and his creation on an immense (if this is the proper adjective) scale. I put my belief in the

[15] The distinction between different kinds of prayer is completely abstract: asking, offering, adoring. There are jealous, selfish, interested demands which are admirable testimonies, beautiful examples of worship. On the other hand, there are avaricious adorations.

world, and this absolute credit is itself my assurance, my certainty, my knowledge — an eschatological knowledge, a knowledge of totality, a knowledge of the future in the present. I put my money on God. This brings immediately to mind the famous contradiction in terms found in Pascal's wager, as though putting my money on God were the same as putting my money on a good horse (of course, the good horse here is the "infinite" one). Betting on a horse is not putting confidence in anyone; it is calculating one's chances. But here we are in an entirely different domain; we are putting our confidence in a Person. We are believing in, confiding in, that Person. We are not believing something; we are believing someone.

If we state this in rational terms, this crediting doubtlessly appears as an act of defiance, illogical, a contradiction, a paradox, folly, an infinite risk, as Kierkegaard has said. But these excessive, intense terms are an expression, on the other extreme, of a dialogue in simplicity itself, in the extraordinary climate of the "fear of God," of infinite distance in infinite proximity.

Seen from our human angle, it is blind obstinacy, an obstinate refusal to see the facts as they are — fanaticism, prescientific or prelogical blindness. It is shocking, irritating, pitiful; it provokes repulsion or admiration, "admiration" pronounced with a fatherly, protective tone of voice. Is not a particular courage, a special heroism, necessary to be able to deny, with all the stubbornness of a boy straight from the farm, evidence that is right in front of our nose?

No, this courage comes from a simple confidence, because it is founded on the *presence* of God. It is a very particular presence, we must grant, since it allows that distance, that fear, that disquiet, that torture caused by absence, those doubts burned into our hearts by the silence of God. But it is a presence just as concrete as that of a spouse, a child — even more alive when it is missing. But it is still a presence, and its supernatural quality does not hinder its naturalness, its "but of course" quality. It is like a long life of getting accustomed, a married couple getting used to each other, a man getting the feel of his trade. For a person new to the trade, the least act, the most familiar movement, seems to be a difficult victory. Nevertheless, it is "just natural." The paradox is only a paradox in the eyes of the stranger and in the language used in speaking to him — *and we are all that stranger, and we are all that believer.*

It is the stranger in us who speaks to the believer in us with the language of absolute risk, lost without a compass on the face of the black ocean: Kierkegaard the stranger speaks to Kierkegaard the believer. So we are double, one of us trying to get the truth across to the other — mysterious for ourselves, unknown to ourselves. The presence of God is perhaps just that. It appears to us to be extraordinary, suspicious, something to be verified, to be doubted, not to be trusted, in any case, a paradox. *This is what we call a mystery*. And so "mystery" means for us what is inexhaustibly unfathomable and what illuminates everything else: obscurity and light.

If, therefore, we speak *to the stranger in us* in the language of hope, we will be speaking the language of folly, of paradox. I put my confidence in the world, in spite of every appearance, in spite of everything. Not only do I place my confidence, but I act accordingly. It is more than an intellectual "wager"; it is an involvement of my entire life. I assume responsibility (heroically, fanatically, *the stranger will say)* for looking at present evil with the eyes of the future, with the prophetic vision of last events, with the look of hope. Such a vision is dialectical, if one ever existed (to use a vocabulary today understood by all), because it exists in reference to a totality, in which we might say that the end precedes the beginning.

Such a totalizing vision, such an assurance concerning the future and eternity (not only in the sense of what is *beyond* time, but as the *absoluteness of here and now),* is only possible in a religious tradition and doctrine. Those who make fun by accusing Christians of "putting money in the bank of heaven," putting aside a tidy little sum as good, selfish savers, are both mistaken and right. A savings account on the other side is the psychosociological interpretation of a spiritual and theological reality. It is true that faith procures an "assurance" (a certitude) that is an "insurance" (policy). It is true that when we credit the Father with our confidence in the covenant, we bring to mind the "credit" of the commercial banks. It is also true that the faith of most believers goes no further than this sociological vulgarization of God's collaboration with man. Perhaps by a certain lapse of our own being (the stranger, I called him above), we make no progress beyond this rough interpretation; let us not forget that the people paid attention only to the healings and predictions. The savings account on the other side belongs to the domain of our love of the marvelous, on the level of myth and sorcery. Every religion drags its weight of selfishness and mythology. Thus in the ore of human nature may be found two natures and two faces of *self-interest* and *love.*

But this savings account on the other side, this insurance policy, and this credit are expressions of a spiritual reality which is hope itself, which depends explicitly on a Word of God, on an assurance given by God, his confiding in us, his revelation (not only the one found in the Bible, but that which is both before and after the Bible's influence on our lives, one that reaches us from within ourselves, a present revelation, contemporaneous and always new, the very presence of the Father).

Hope is faith in the Word of God. Not that word which he *once* entrusted to his people, but that word made incarnate in his Son, which is still living. Christ is God's present, daily revelation, the daily food for hope.

A meditation on Christ is absolutely indispensable for a meditation on evil. For Christ is the incarnation of the future in the present, of *that anticipation which constitutes almost the speciality of the "knowledge" we call hope.* Christ could be considered the here-and-now witness whom we are permitted to "use as a witness" at every moment. He is the concrete and living anticipation of God's designs for creation. He is eternity which has moved into a *before* and *after,* an *after* incarnate in *before,* a reversal of time because eternity has come in (if intervention, which implies a given moment, and eternity may be united; this is, however, the paradox of reality itself). The tendentious expression "a savings account in eternity" expresses a horizontal space without perspective, space with only two psychological dimensions, a brutal and magnificent reality which the Apostle Paul, for one, was not afraid (for he was not so delicate as some who do not want to contaminate themselves) to call an *earnest* (earnest money given as guarantee for an agreement). The Son was given by the Father as the guarantee of his covenant, an earnest made up of living flesh renewed daily. This earnest, which nourishes our hope, is that he loves us, that he desires something for us; he wants to do something with his creation, including what we judge and suffer and call *evil.*

Such an assurance, founded on such credit, offers the two contradictory (for the rationalist) aspects of folly and prudence, of a risk that might be costly and a sure investment. We oscillate from one to the other when we pass by unaware of the source whence these contradictory appearances, these shadow figures, derive.

In the same way, the simple workingman's faith and the *credo quia absurdum* are expressions close to the basic hope which they betray or denature and which gives them an element of truth.

This hope does, in fact, belong both to folly and to reason, to confidence in someone and to a theological doctrine, to individual proof and to community tradition. It also belongs both to knowledge and to action: it is praxis. It is passivity and activity, extreme docility in taking and extreme provocation in demanding, both acceptance and struggle. It is that very attitude which we might call *political* in the very midst of suffering and disease. I will come back to this point.

Extreme passivity linked with extreme activity – only some saints may achieve so high a goal. The action which originates in us is God's action by us, within us. Even in my action, I receive everything. My combat is obedience. In my most personal creativity, in my most personal initiatives, I am an instrument in the hands of the Creator. I am a vase, always ready to receive, an ear ready to listen, an arm always ready to serve. Even in my work, even in my anger and revolt, when I kick back in anger, hope is yet in me like a deeper docility, one even more permanent than my movements of anxiety or temper. Some speak of a voluntary attitude in cases where a more penetrating eye would see complete surrender; they speak of cowardly resignation in cases where every energy is gathered for the struggle. These "activist" attitudes are really only surrenders, resignations, active only in order to make themselves appear important and to gain personal prestige. True activity does not appear to every eye from its inception; years pass while it slowly sprouts until one day a tree shadows us with its fullness. Hope lives with the long, slow life of plant growth; we would only have to change the speed of projection and its slow sprouting would become a vast display of fireworks. But our myopia misses its movement far away on another time scale before which our hasty comings and goings lose patience and die a death with no tomorrow.

Hope is a fertilized fertility. In pain, it rises like bread. We are dough kneaded by God. It hurts when he kneads the dough which he will make into bread. The seed dies in the earth and then grows up into an immense tree. Pain is perhaps the sign that we must die to ourselves in order to be united with creation.

Hope Springs from Pain

We must die in order to be healed. Repeating the accents of a Kierkegaard, Neher discovers in Jeremiah the greatest joy even in the depths of despair:

> *It is from the depths of this time that Jacob will be saved.* Not by leaving this time of anguish, but by penetrating deeper into it, into its very substance,

into its abyss of nothingness. . . . Healing (is) in the gaping, burning wound. Edification is in abounding ruin. Approach to God is in retreat. . . . Thus the length of exile is also redemption. . . .[16]

Hope does not endeavor to escape the cruel present in order to find refuge in better times; it does not flee forward in what is really only headlong retreat. It does not seek refuge; it settles down at the heart of evil and from it extracts joy. But hope does not rejoice in evil by a kind of repugnant masochism; nor does it refuse to count on the future, the promises of tomorrow. Hope does not abandon the conflict with today's suffering. Neither does it see the best in the worst; nor does it believe that God is able to make the worst into the best — but its joy bursts forth from the wound itself, a bitter joy made of tears mixed with love. Yes, we know that it is possible to laugh and to cry at the same time, to be immersed in both happiness and pain. But this is not some psychological blend of joy and suffering; they cannot be mixed because they are not of the same order. Joy does not alternate with suffering, is not mixed with it; it comes out of it like blood from an open wound, in a kind of bursting forth, of absolute liberation, an absolute, eternity in the present. "Freed, freed from everything, freed from the last bond tying me to the earth. I'm free, Brand, free!" (Ibsen). Not *everything* as a recompense for nothing, according to him, but in the depths of *nothing* is to be found everything. It is living experience, by no means a dream or empty words. Hope is not only a category of the future, nor is it a category of the future in the present. It is the category of an instant, that is, of eternity. Hope may be defined as a present joy, a joy in the present, a present fullness, belonging to the present and in the present. The material of which it is made is pain — a matter which does not wear out. When joy is made from pain, "nothing is being risked." It is a good investment. "There is a chance; there is faith." So true is this that the hero's security may closely resemble that of the ambushed villain. The champion of faith, says Kierkegaard in *Fear and Trembling,* is the common man, and nothing but an imperceptible nuance separates him from the small, down-to-earth interests of the common man; nevertheless, his is another world, he is free.

Hope: A Community Initiative for the Birth of the World

Hope is the other name for liberty.

But we would be wrong if we saw in it a completely developed

[16] Andre Neher, *Jeremie* [Jeremiah] (Paris: Librairie Plon), p. 197.

liberty, stopped in the satisfaction of that instant which is eternity. Hope is the fullness of the present biting into the future, into a world ready to be born, into the end of time which it includes in its grasp, which it encompasses with one fell swoop.

Just as contemplation may not be excluded from action, so hope is able to make knowledge and participation identical, to see in this action an unceasing confirmation of knowledge, and knowledge a confirmation of action. By acting, I know. By obtaining this knowledge, I contribute to accomplishment itself, to the transformation of the world. *Such is the identity of testimony and hope.*

We said concerning the prophet that his docility is nevertheless a pressing *question* which leaves God no rest. He listens and proclaims the word *of* Yahweh, but he proclaims *to* Yahweh the words of his creature. He listens; he bends his ear to God's word. But he also possesses; he demands; he gets God to listen to him. He is ear and mouth. He has both God's ear and God's mouth. And God's ear and mouth are turned toward the world; they work history; they are harnessed to the work of childbirth.

Thus hope is not content with smiling expectation, confident in the happy conclusion of the trial. *Hope is travail.* Hope waits, which means that it is working for creation in childbirth. It is not only liberated; it is liberating. Hope is attached to the world's pain like a worker to his tool, a tool no longer dangerous for his calloused hands. Hope is worked pain, transformed, denied pain. Both of them work together and tie a knot of fruitful negation. Hope espouses pain with a loving but mortal embrace — not a deadly embrace, but creative, as the artist espouses his marble and denies its existence as marble, and the marble dies in the work he takes from it.

Pain can receive no explanation, or rather no meaning, except in a perspective of dialectic and liberty.

Pain takes on meaning through our *negation* (as Hegel would understand negation) of pain. And liberty is this conquest of the universe by man, his effort to deny nature as it is, to transcend, and to transform it. Pain *is,* to the extent that it is denied by man, by his work, and by his hope. It has no consistency except through our negation. It assumes the form of our grasp, of our imprint on the world, like two wrestlers whose bodies mold each other. Pain *is* to the extent that it is not, as today's lovers of the paradox would say, which means that it *is* to the extent that it is transcended, to the extent that it becomes an instrument of our liberation, of our liberty. Pain is *meaning,* and this meaning must go through the phase of meaninglessness. So denying any meaning to evil is affirming it. It is not by saying yes, yes, that the world will be made to progress. The one who says *no* is also in his own way contributing to its progress, although he may deny it vigorously.

The word negation (as in "denying") has a double meaning, but negation/revolt does not appear to us to be so different, nor really much less fruitful than negation/transcendence. Revolt is one form, and not the least important, of transcendence; it is its first phase, the most painful, that of disestablishment and woe. Revolt, which denies evil any meaning, works toward the birth of that meaning. It cooperates. Negative negation and positive negation can scarcely be called two phases, or two complementary persons. We realize that they are two appearances of a single motor force in history. The refusal to advance has only the appearance of immobility; it is really a tension, a haste, an effective effort which adds its weight to the apparently angelic work of others. When viewed from the standpoint of the communion of the saints in unity, it may be seen that it is all one common effort.

For hope, just as it is situated in the totality of history, takes in the community of men and is incapable of separating any one man's effort from that of the community. Its eye is able to discern within the most contradictory, the most baffling attitudes, a fruitful contribution to the effort. The beatific establishment of one, the porcine indifference of another, meanness, pride, revolt, and refusal – hope does not reject them as useless materials, tares to be burned. There are, however, tares to be burned, according to the Gospel: metaphysical wickedness is indefensible, and separation from God is death. Otherwise, would hell have any meaning?

But the challenge thrown out by hope is the fact that it believes in mortal sin but does not stop there; it does not want to believe in it. It does not want to stop there. Nothing is ever terminated or definitively closed; the moment is never reached when all the cards are on the table as long as history is not ended, as long as the effort of one is inseparable from that of the others, as long as the blend is so fine that it would take a very crafty eye to discern the contribution of one from the refusal to collaborate of another.

How is that? Has not God proclaimed that he will separate his creatures one by one according to their works, and is not the logical conclusion that each person decides his own destruction or salvation? This appears to be indubitable; yet it is still true that hope is flawless solidarity among created beings. What I do contributes to the salvation of someone else, just as what he does contributes to my own. But the manner is incomprehensible and does not exclude the judgment of God, while it still permits the intervention of hope into judgment. My refusal to act is perhaps a more fruitful way of acting. Who can fathom the intentions and effects of our actions? Who can fathom the mystery of this solidarity which unites us into a single mass nonetheless made up of personal freedoms? Who can fathom the communion of the saints? We can say it exists, but we cannot say how. We can say that it does not contradict the infinite singularity of each person, his liberty as concerns his own destruction and salvation. But we cannot say how to surmount such a contradiction.

Hope is the experience of active participation, effective, renewed daily within the community—participation in the birth of the world, one whose purpose is to form a common effort, to become itself a part of that effort, to unite men in history, and to unify history.

Finally, hope lives from an assurance of the future based on an event which has already taken place and which sums it all up: the resurrection. The theology of hope is identical with the theology of the resurrection, that is, with faith in the lordship of Christ, present and alive in history.

"If Christ has not been raised, your faith is futile. . . ." (1 Corinthians 15:17) ; such is the identity of hope and the resurrection.

Our task is obviously not to treat here the fact itself, the spiritual event called resurrection. Our only reason for bringing it in is to emphasize its identity with the content, the body of hope.

Hope, as many have emphasized, "is a moment of truth" (P. Ganne) . For to the extent that it is an event inscribed in the totality of history, it attains an order of reality more concrete, more real, than that of a simple observation of the present event, isolated from its contest. "I put them back in hope, by putting them back into the truth of history" *(Ibid.)*.

Hope is a dialectic of the present and the future, of the instant and eternity. It situates us with respect to the future and calls us to that future. It is knowledge, a motor force.

Finally, hope brings us to the condition of adult man, capable of realizing the totality of his relations in the world and within history. Hoping is becoming a part of a solidarity, of a tradition.

Part 3
Conclusion

The Suppression of Pain

Time, Liberty, Work

In the light of the preceding considerations, the relationship between *pain* and *time,* mentioned several times in the course of this study, changes both as to dimension and meaning.

When we speak of time — not the false, abstract time of our calculations, but living duration as we live it out — some think of time as the rhythms of nature, biological and cosmological — seasons, generations, geological or solar periods. Others refer to the time of memory and of man's history. A third category separates neither this memory and history nor the cosmic and biological rhythms from the growth of creation still advancing toward its fulfillment. True time is eschatological time (that is, made meaningful through the notion of "the end of time").

Becoming has, therefore, two accepted meanings: the *flow* of time belongs to natural time; *fulfillment* belongs, if I may say so, to supernatural time, that is, to the time of history, of the spirit, whether understood in a strictly religious sense or not.

A Time for Atheism and a Time for Faith

Rather than two kinds of time, these are two ways of looking at time. That time called "natural" time, which appears as a perpetual beginning again, a cyclical becoming, or an involution toward the stability of a dead equilibrium; time as understood in mechanical physics, but also as understood by Heraclitean, Nietzschean, or Sivaitean thought — all these conceptions of time are expressions of an atheistic metaphysical outlook on time, or stated in another way, a manner of living time as an aging, a degradation toward death. It is our atheism of word or deed that makes time endless and senseless. Time offers this facet to the one who looks on as a nonparticipating, unconcerned spectator.

Cyclical or involutionary time is an expression of quarantined time, time separated from our great adventure (rather, our way of separating ourselves from that adventure).

Time which gets nowhere is only *a (negative) category of human faith,* which does not know, which cannot and does not desire to know (understand, be born with, walk along with) time, true time, creative time.

"Natural" time is therefore the absence of love.

The time of "ever returning" is an expression of hell for us, of our lack of confidence in the fulfillment of a universal plan. It is a viewpoint, a form of pessimism, an unhappy state of consciousness.

On the other hand, time directed like a vector, which "stretches out its neck" (Apostle Paul) toward the end of the race, with one goal only, one hope only, one ascendance, and one effort toward one fulfillment, one becoming, becoming what I am, one realization of the calling inscribed in man and the universe: this time is that belonging to faith, and (as in an encounter with faith) it is that of revelation.

Time, Biological Growth, and History

Having reminded ourselves of this relationship, must we dwell in a relative state of "viewpoints"? By no means.

Involution, degradation, and man's eternal beginning again are all striking confirmations of the "powers of diminution" (Teilhard de Chardin), and they may be seen in everything that is differentiated and degraded, which returns to the nothingness of this world. Man "returns to the dust." Cataclysms of cosmic proportions, inhuman nature, the bright sun shining on the disaster brought on by hard rain — these romantic themes are no less less true when treated in poetic form. Pain belongs to this senselessness of time, blind to the spirit, deaf to demands, to hope, to human faithfulness; it marches indifferently on with its Sivaite gait, and leaves man lost in the immensity of the world.

But, and this is a paradox which belies this senselessness of the time of death and evil, *two stupefying facts* arise, which are and are not on the same order, two facts which arouse our astonishment by being associated with each other and by very obviously confirming each other.

1. "Eternity" is in me (in my mind), and with all its strength it judges, transcends, and denies the existence of "wasted time." My mind (my eternity) transforms raw time into history. If raw time existed alone, nameless and faceless, without a goal and without

an end, then the impossibility of negating it (if I may say so) would be a part of its own existence. There is no history, says Jean Lacroix, for a purely historical being (that is, immersed in raw time).

Now, history is a part of my consciousness; it dominates it, unifies it, both denies and fulfills it, names it, speaks of it – such is time.

2. What is extraordinary is that this meaningful time, which is a part of my consciousness, is shown to be at work also in the things of this world. It may be seen in all the forms of growth, of differentiation, of "complexification" (Teilhard de Chardin) in biological time.

These material facts, so lowly in their daily renewal, are so uncontestable as to be barely noticeable: the growth of an embryo is an act of *construction*. It produces (induces) a more differentiated state from a less differentiated state. There is no need of a theory dealing with evolution to accept that, whether from a finalistic or causalistic point of view.

I was saying that there is an astonishing encounter, a mutual confirmation between history as it is inscribed in my consciousness and the creative evolution inscribed in things (in the spirit of things).

So the word is out; there is spirit in things, history in things, spirit and meaning in time itself.

The identity of liberty and history consists in *moving* out of time, in *making* time.

Man does, of course, possess the power to use time to make time, the power of transforming, taming, domesticating time – like a horse or a wild elephant – of putting time to work, of making time into work, a working time. Time becomes a *work!*

But, on the other hand, is it not a ridiculous claim to believe that our sole mastery of time may transform an indifferent line into a vector, an arrow, growth, work – do we not see life itself at work, edifying, differentiating, defying death?

Does time belong to life? Or is it a monopoly of human consciousness? Time, with all the depth of growth, of an embryogenesis, belongs to the world before or at the same time that it belongs to human consciousness. That is why biological pain belongs to time before it is called "suffering" by civilized man. The individual does not make life; he makes history.[1] This is doubtlessly true, but man's

[1] Binswanger, *Rêve et existence* [Dream and existence] (Paris: Desclée de Brouwer), p. 192.

historical time rises out of earthly time and appears as both adhesion and negation, *yes* and *no,* time as confirmation and time as opposition (inopportune time).

Our spirit, creator of time, participates in the spirit which is in things. It recognizes both its dependence and its emancipation (with regard to the spirit of things).

And man's memory is separated from the memory of the things of life, in order to become transfigured into a conscious memory of itself, capable not only of conserving and living the past over again, but also of bringing the past into the present, of "presentifying" it as the past, of dating and naming it.

The Identity of Faith, Life, and Time

This "time found again," which means that it has significance, verified in an embryo by the scientist, edified in turn by my consciousness into history, into a civilization, into education [2] — this is exactly what affirms faith. This is why Marxism is a religion (in a positive sense). For Marxism, *history does exist;* that is, the world has meaning (in the double sense of the term) and a termination.

The simplest and most basic intuition of any religious faith is that "there is meaning"; time is, in fact, time and not an illusion, a maya.

The Pavlovian scientist, the most confirmed believer in causality, in determinism, in "materialism," has stopped obeying the dictates of causality as soon as he recognizes in man's "brain" the power of making history ("revolution"). This is what we call dialectics (Hegel, Marx): a dialogue, a factor in the transformation of the world, a dialogue between my "causes" (my predecessors, my origins, my conditioning) and the finality of man's take-over of our destiny. We are constantly bounced back and forth between the reflection of dialectics in ideology and human consciousness as the driving force in history.

With regard to man's destiny, Marxism is less deterministic than ancient man (who was apparently more religious, but the fantasy of the gods gives fatality a face; nothing belongs to the human worker — with the exception of Hercules), than the Buddhist, for whom time is maya.

What difference, then, is there between biblical faith and that secular faith called "atheistic"? The first type recognizes and proclaims what the second does not recognize or proclaim. The Marxist

[2] For the role of the school, cf. J. Lacroix, *L'Ecole et la nation* [The school and the nation], Journées universitaires de Reims (April 16, 1962).

takes over his own destiny, but literally, without knowing why. For if history may be reduced to raw time, it moves into nothingness; it is devoted to nothingness; it is nothingness. Even more, how can we account for the fact that we have ever conceived of the idea of and the requirement for making history?

Religious faith goes to the very end, as it were, of Marxist "logic." If I have endowed my destiny with a meaning (a history), if this destiny can in fact (not in an illusory or temporary way) receive its historical status, it must not be lost in nothingness. Man's time must be included in the growth of the world.

It has been said that the *death* of the individual or of humanity provides the fatal snare for Marxism.

Every atheist at work on the earth (the Marxist, Camus, every man in his own way) resembles an insect, or a living embryo, working at a task of which he does not see the totality, the meaning. So it is with instinct: It has spirit, but does not have a spirit; it pursues an end, without naming that end. The materialist, whatever name he may give himself, also contributes to the edification of a work in which he does not want to believe. For there is no work which is not total, which is not part of a totality.

Eternity is essential to the notion of work (this is why every creator has desired eternity because he knows that man's work is, for all appearances, perishable). Death devitalizes the notion of work, reduces it to nothingness. The death of each one of us is a daily verification of that horrible truth. It cruelly belies our work, everything that makes up our being, everything that we are.

When Heidegger asserted that man is a being-for-death, that death is the sign of man, he thrust his knife into the weakest spot — but he is right, for only man appears capable of grasping death as such. The idea of nothingness, Bergson has said, is a pseudo-idea fabricated from being, which was supposed to have been removed by thought. Does death not *realize* before our eyes this mad operation? In fact, it only realizes it in order to be capable of annihilating it. The animal does not die; death is death only for man, who is therefore a being-for-death.

Thus, paradoxically, when Heidegger says that man is a being-for-death, by these words he is designating man's meaning in life.

Only a being for whom life is *life,* for whom time is *time* (history, meaning, work), only such a being is capable of knowing death.

And death only exists for the being capable of denying death with all his strength.

Man, as we might sum up Heidegger's words, is the being-for-life, that is, for whom there is meaning, history, work. It is the same thing as saying that man is the being-for-faith (or hope), that he is a religious being.

Faith is hidden in the least of our acts. However, it is not hidden like the least of biological functions (embryogenesis, or instinct) which is, as it were, transcended by itself, but in our liberty, in our own realization of the notion of work, of history, of totality.

There is a very real identity between what we call an act of faith and the notion and demand for totality. Unless he commits suicide, man works as though he were contributing to an overall work. And this is true whether he asserts it or denies it, whether he knows it or is ignorant of it (after the fashion of an insect which is a meticulous worker in contributing to a totality which he cannot see).

Recognizing that voluntarily or not I am working in terms of a totality is pronouncing the word *creation,* is voluntarily or not showing myself to be a religious being.

Speaking out our faith is attaining the lucid frankness of admitting that we believe in the reality of time, in the reality of work, because they are part of a totality without which neither time nor work would have any meaning. If I were to put all my efforts into denying this meaning, mankind and I (and the very work I would construct in order to demonstrate the vanity of time would be there to belie me, as a magnet betrays itself by its attracting force) would only be proclaiming the meaning of work and time.

There are individuals who resemble insects; by every one of their actions so admirably full of meaning they sing out (in spite of themselves) the reality of time and of creation.

Revelation meets and supports reason and confirms the consistency of the time of creation. God works naturally and supernaturally to make us participate in his plan for us. We would have contributed to it anyhow, but he wants us to collaborate intelligently. This knowledge of God's plan is called covenant, alliance; but its secular name is consciousness, liberty, sense of history, sense of death, the power of vanquishing death.

The Transmutation of Pain: Pain as Time

This knowledge of time as being meaningful, as the sign of a creation in the process of becoming, of moving toward a future, in childbirth, must obviously change pain itself.

I must admit that my knowledge of death and time (memory

and imagination) augments pain, literally creates it as pain, as we have already said, and prolongs pain, giving it infinite dimensions.

But I will add that pain, like death, is transcended by that knowledge; pain is converted, as it were. It is referred to a *pain on the other side* without which pain itself would in fact be dissolved, but without disappearing. This other side of pain does not dissolve pain; it suppresses it, denies it.

The knowledge of pain – that is, of time – both creates pain and suppresses it. But it can stop in the midst of its progress and pathologically excite to bursting that which is yet incapable of taking upon itself the meaning conferred upon it.

Work is the means given to us to suppress pain, that is, to perform both a clinical and a spiritual transmutation. Work, like any practical act, denies the abstract duality of what is produced (in the organism) and its theoretical meaning. It brings about the synthesis of empiricism (as a physician sees it in a patient who has *gone back to work,* who has been reeducated to work) and theory.

The physician and suffering men will doubtlessly rise up in revolt, because we are incapable of doing with pain as we please. We may work all we want; we may cooperate in meaningfulness, create meaning, but this does not bring an end to pain as such. Some believe that this is a good demonstration of the difference between pain and evil (or suffering).

In fact, I must repeat, that pain which is most directly physical is open to transformation by meaning, by time.

I would object strenuously to anyone's imagining that I am somehow giving short shrift to certain intolerable pains, which we all put all of our strength and faculties into trying to heal! But such an emergency situation hardly puts us into the best situation for meditation and searching on a deeper and different plane.

We could, as other civilizations have done and are doing, become master over our pain, but on a deeper level, at the very roots of civilization, in the way we are affected by events, time, burns, and wounds. Master over our pain, master over death. When the meaning of pain changes, so does its intensity. So it is with the soldier in battle, or with a Buddhist priest who burns himself to death in Saigon. We must avoid letting ourselves be influenced by the prestige of our own daily experience in our own civilization if we wish to launch into a theory of the connections between pain and time.

Pain becomes pain when it is espoused by time, and by the same act the status of pain becomes that of the problem of evil.

That is why in our human experience pain and evil are identical; all of evil passes into us by way of *pain/time* (as some speak of *space / time*).

Transforming Pain by Work:
Both Recognizing It and Suppressing It

We must be able to understand pain as part of a total picture in which the world is transformed by work. The world is about to give birth; its pangs are pain. It gives birth to joy in the *suppression* of pain. The vocabulary of Hegel and Marx here comes back to the vocabulary of faith. Pain stands out like mileposts in the alienation of mankind by nature and society. And the suppression of this alienation is at the heart of a final reconciliation of man with nature and society. Productive work characterizes both man's pain [3] and his victorious effort to overcome pain. It also characterizes God's interruption and intervention in history and the universe. This passage from Neher's work on Jeremiah strikingly illustrates what we have been saying: "Work. An astonishing, unexpected term which is nevertheless the only one conceivable since Jeremiah himself uses it to define God's presence in history (Jeremiah 50:25): *'The Lord of Hosts has a work to do in Chaldea.' Melacha* in Hebrew." [4] Work means both creative liberation *(melacha)* and working service *(avoda). Childbirth* is *pain,* but at the same time it manifests the most astonishing creation of liberty and life – a new being joins the race.

Man's liberating work is identical with the childbirth. Work is the travail of God's creation, in pain, and in the suppression of pain. Pain is only comprehensible when viewed in a context of liberation, of liberty.

The strange relationship between liberty and evil, which I wrote about in 1950 (here quoted on p. 176), is that man's liberty must assume the weight of evil. Liberty cannot be imputed with evil because it alone is capable of bearing it, even of transforming the world. I wanted nothing to do with pain as a scapegoat. I did and still do believe in a liberty capable of putting the weight of its initiative, of its work, on the scales of the balance. The suppression of evil is *action, practical action.* It is not an idea, but a work.

The suppression of pain and the recognition of its value, its

[3] The etymology of the French word for work, *travail: tripalus* (the prods used to keep oxen in line); *tripaliare* (to torture). During the middle ages an executioner was called a *travailleur* (a worker). Compare J. Lacroix, *op. cit.*

[4] Andre Neher, *Jeremie* [Jeremiah] (Paris: Librairie Plon), p. 178.

dignity, are one and the same act. I must not treat again the "dialectic" of work and illness which I have studied elsewhere.[5] Illness, pain, and evil are the inexhaustible materials for our enterprise of transforming, of humanizing, and of deifying the world. They are also the ever-receding horizon, the *over there* of that transformation which situates it and gives its setting. Evil is *beyond* man's creative activity, not only as an ever-receding limit, but especially as a reminder, a sign intended for us, which puts our creative activity into the hands of the Creator, as a grace received from him.

Accepting and Not Accepting

Evil must therefore both be recognized and suppressed. *And recognizing it is exactly the same thing as suppressing it.* This is a truth for the suffering individual, a truth for underdeveloped people. The beginning of the healing of pain is in this recognition; the *attention* of my eye fixed on it, which respects pain in the one bearing it and joins his combat against it. Transforming my pain by someone else's presence is a curious psychological and sociological problem which brings me back to the beginning of this study (pp. 13 ff., 21 ff). Yes, the presence of some people changes pain into a comical and lamentable superfetation, but this happens because this presence itself provided, either maliciously or stupidly, the possibility and the temptation. In such a case the deficient quality of the presence must be examined. A presence either at the extreme of suspicious indifference or at the opposite extreme of pusillanimous solicitude causes exaggeration, becomes an accomplice of pain. But another kind of presence destroys pain with solitude, furnishing arms both to combat pain and to accept it.

We suffer less when we are not alone. This leads to one form of healing by love (the other form is furnished by the very contents of its initiative: work, material help, added energy). This is true in the individual (has not psychoanalysis rediscovered that frustrated love leads to a great many unbalanced states?) and is true for people. The third world is hungry, and it is hungry for recognition. Justice is the symbol of this synthesis of recognition and material help. Love is another face of food, merchandise, industry, education of students and technicians. A nation of people no more puts up with paternalistic compassion than does an individual. Such compassion, I said before, incites and suggests complaining

[5] Jacques Sarano, *Essai sur la signification du corps,* p. 115. English edition is *The Meaning of the Body* (Philadelphia: The Westminster Press, 1966).

by the one who lacks virility. *Solidarity* realizes that synthesis of the recognition and suppression of evil and shares the single bread of bitterness and liberation.

Some will call this synthesis contradictory; one aspect of it grants full citizenship and sanctuary to the evil that the other is driving out. But this objection arises only on the level of intellectual antinomies. For example, examine the following contradiction, so banal that it adds to the pathos of everyday life: "We must, so it seems, do battle with pain as long as we are able and accept it (as a kind of trial or mysterious good) when we cannot win." Examine this abstract division, terribly false, between a portion of pain considered as an arm for the living being, another portion as a harmful beast to be destroyed, with a third and final form (the ugliest, what is "left over," which no one knows how to accommodate), as that which must be accommodated as a trial.

But this horrible division disappears as soon as we consent to "thaw" a problem into praxis, into the transformation of the world and its inhabitants.[6] This is the same pain which I have accepted

[6] Teilhard de Chardin devotes some pages to evil ("passivities of diminution") in *Le milieu divin* (Paris: Editions du Seuil, 1957), pp. 80ff; English edition is *The Divine Milieu,* (New York: Harper & Row, Publishers, 1960). These pages hardly seem convincing as explanations; they must be understood as an exhortation, a "praxis," often as a *prayer.* This is why it seems useless to me to stop at the *letter* of his distinction between "a first time" of struggle (pp. 87, 97) and a second time of acceptation. Nor must we spend too much time with the old saws which Teilhard takes up: God struggles *with us* (p. 86)—a very mediocre help ("God *can not* . . ., the present state of creation *does not enable him to* . . ." (p. 89). As a skillful sculptor he is able to turn "evil into good" (p. 90). We fall, while we await the definitive victory of good over evil, like soldiers who will never see the great peace to which they have contributed by their death (p. 89). (This reminds us of the Marxists, blamed for sacrificing one or two generations for the benefit of the great upheaval to come.)

All this would be ridiculous *if Teilhard's great prayer did not transfigure it.* Evil is a sign that we must die to ourselves in order to become better able to unite with God (pp. 92–93). "In all of these somber hours, God, grant that I might understand that it is thou (if only my faith is strong enough) who art painfully separating the fibers of my being in order to penetrate to the very marrow of my existence, in order to carry me away in thyself" (p. 95). No longer is it a question of accepting what we cannot conquer, but of promoting with a single loving gesture the "natural personalization of man and his supernatural depersonalization in Christo" (p. 102), extending to the perfection of a creation in preparation.

This effort, which turns away the sting of death, takes its strength directly from the example, the life, and the resurrection of Christ, who vanquished, in a fashion which we might call experimental, death and evil. And this turning away which we are to accomplish is accomplished by Christ in us, and we participate with him in his victory—the exact opposite of defeat or resignation. Thus the transformation of the world is constantly progressing, and the *destruction of evil* is just that, "destruction."

in combat and which I have accepted to combat. Struggle can be a form, and doubtlessly the proudest form, of obedience. And obedience in turn – if it is not cowardly resignation, surrender, or worse – true obedience to God, is seen in its truest form in struggle. Jacob shows his truest submissive sonship to God in his aggressiveness. In resistance the salt of filial loves does not do away with the joy of tears. "The only true prophet is the man who has obstinately tried to resist God and who has been made full by the defeat he had to suffer." [7]

Yes, it is in *questioning,* as we are constantly discovering to our own astonishment in the Psalms and the prophets, that the dualism between the abhorrence and the acceptance of evil is resolved. In those vehement tones,[8] it at first seems foolish to hear an alternation of invective and happiness.

[7] Neher, *op. cit.,* p. 50.

[8] The solution for the "problem" of evil is passion, as Etienne Borne has so excellently written in his fine study, *Le problème du mal* [The problem of evil] (Paris: Presses Universitaires de France, 1958). *Salvation by passion* "is the narrow path of liberation"; it is action, "polemics," "politics." It has aspects both of Prometheus and of Christ's Passion. I am in full agreement with the author's dialectic, although his virtuosity is sometimes sacrificed to false symmetries (an example of a false political symmetry on p. 115: "an illusory transcendence of democracy toward nationalism or socialism participates in a retrograde movement of the human spirit and compromises the dialectics of liberation. . . .").

I much appreciated the analysis of the wisdom and lucidity in Jewish anti-aesthetic thought, the necessary confrontation of the atheistic phase. I found very correct his emphasis on the unjustifiable, *"unmediatizable"* (p. 21) character of evil—an emphasis occasionally reaching vehemence (pp. 18 ff., the "immorality" of "lying" nature "gives itself the lie"—here I agree not only with the author's thought but with his very words), which some might consider uncalled for.

I would be less decisive in my acceptance of "idealistic discourse" and wisdom. Is there such a thing as an "evil-as-evil" (cf. p. 20) which would be separable from evil-for-us? The *"unmediatizable"* category already belongs to the world of meanings (see in the present study, above, pp. 63ff.).

It is true, finally, that the *problem of evil casts doubt in a very dangerous way on all of philosophy* (pp. 2, 114). But, as I see it, philosophy is to be identified with man's *questionings,* whatever his *a priori* opinions, his inspiration, his methods may be, and this is true even for those men and women who deny philosophy any reality. The contestation and death of philosophy are also philosophy.

It goes beyond the limits of reasoning reason, both as *passion* and as action. Kierkegaard and Marx both contested any value in philosophy, one in passion, the other in action. But paradox, contradiction, and even confusion are all philosophy (whether good or bad is another problem). And on the other hand, beliefs and theologies, which philosophy prudently or disdainfully sets aside, are nourished by philosophy and belong to that permanent questioning by which it is defined. Philosophy, finally, is not only theory but action and history: Hegel brought back to earth is still Hegel, and transforming the world is another way of philosophizing.

Such is the "paradox," says the philosopher in his jargon, or rather the living experience of joy in the midst of suffering itself, extracted from suffering, because of it, in spite of it, by it. Neher's *"nonetheless"* in his *Jérémie* is one such expression of that turning of the tables which we call hope, where God's passion responds superabundantly to the insistent questionings of his creature.[9] "Here I am, your God," in the simultaneousness of my time which is eternity, in the slowness of my haste, in that anger which loves and saves, which constructs in the midst of destruction – here and everywhere God is in history, an untiring traveler, an untiring collaborator, interdependent with his creatures.

Struggling with God is our response to evil and our acceptance of it. And how does God need to struggle with evil? May I refer the gainsayer to the chapter on the intellectual explanations and refutations of evil. We are able to surmount with one movement (according to Bergson, like the hand's movement, so simple in comparison with the hundreds of filings it can produce with one pass) the paltry dualism of acceptance and struggle – of evil and God's love. But such a "synthesis" is practical; it is beyond the scope of rationalistic antinomies. Other personages have come on the stage whose silent obstinacy destroys the massacre in which one after the other, the "scientific status" and the "philosophical status" of pain, perished. The only thing capable of putting arguers in the presence of the accomplished fact that the destruction of evil is now going on is *hope,* man's *action in alliance with God.* Such is history's answer to a problem bogged down in contradictions. Where the contradictor gets bogged down, the witness, the man of testimony, cuts straight through the knot of problems and provides proof by his own deed and example, overcomes more than he explains – and then follows on beyond.

One's answer to the problem of evil is embodied in history, in a history, temporal/eternal history, as Péguy would say. Christ taught us about evil through his own experience when he *realized* a meaning in pain, not as a payment or a buying back, but a redeeming example, a testimony. After Job, the Cross provides us with a second parable of pain and evil, but infinitely more searching because it was lived out, because it was completely vanquished, *destroyed* by the Resurrection.

Thus, our destruction of evil can only be an imitation. The Gordian knot may be cut by a created being only on the condition that he permits everything to be done to and through him while

[9] Neher, *op. cit.,* pp. 204–218.

he does everything by himself; the knot resists that hand which wants to do *everything* by itself. The most obstinate work, if it forgets that the ripening of history only belongs to God, short-circuits itself, halts all communication and progress by its own noise. Our self-sufficiency halts any progress in intellectual problems by making them into subtle antinomies, by making the problems of life into alternatives with no tomorrow.[10] God's silence, as Paul Tournier has so finely written, is the noise we make with all our dilemmas: "While we ask God questions which go unanswered, he is always asking us others to which we give no heed." And the answer comes in a way that we were not expecting: by the change in that situation which brought on our silence, our readiness to listen to God.[11] This transformation and this maturation have modified the very "data" of the dilemma which we wanted to force open like a stuck lock; they provided the key, resolved the contradiction which held us up as long as we were opposing terms mutually exclusive and outside the limits of each other. Only by a more profound study can the dilemma of struggle and acceptance be resolved, and the same is true of that struggle between the recognition and the destruction of evil: "Give me a heart to hear and to *administer* thy people." These words of Solomon contain the practical synthesis which is to work until the end of time for the destruction of evil and the establishment of good, of beatitude, of the kingdom of God.

[10] Paul Tournier, *Tenir tête ou céder* (Geneva: Labor et Fides, 1962); English edition is *To Resist or to Surrender?* (Richmond: John Knox Press, 1964). This small volume is a model of simplicity, psychological finesse, and spiritual profundity.

[11] "We cannot even wait to be sure that we have heard God's voice before obeying, *for it is from obedience to obedience that we learn better to listen to God." Ibid.,* p. 54. (italics author's).

Afterword

Pain, evil: these are two names for a single problem. Or rather, evil is problem pain. This problem is not one of man's problems among others, as we might be led to believe by the writings of most philosophers, but *the* problem, the reality without which *there would be no problem,* no problem of life, no problem of knowledge. These problems only take up in different areas the same problem, the same questioning.

If philosophy is essentially questioning, questioning is born of contrariety.

My starting point was pain as contradiction. I was not content to make only a nomenclature of different kinds of pain or a juxtaposition of "normal" and "abnormal" pain, useful or harmful pain, but, as is done in a courtroom confrontation, I set the contradictions of pain over against one another. This was the first step in resolving the problem.

Evil originates necessarily and exclusively in this contrariety in pain: If we destroy, not pain, but the *yes/no* of pain, the problem of evil does not even appear.

This is why evil hangs from my study of pain like an enormous appendix. It would be impossible to detach it (to make of it a separate study) without emasculating the intention and the vigor of the approach to pain that I have chosen – as the choice is made to do battle on a given terrain. The contradictions of pain cause us to think of evil; such is their function. The problem of evil hangs like a lead weight attached to the foot of pain.

The second part, a study of evil, takes up a progressive investigation divided into three chapters.

First, the notion of evil is not immediate; it may not be grasped in its essence, without an analysis (an endless analysis) of all the presuppositions, of all the implications without which evil is never born into the world – without these it would end in a miscarriage!

Because they skip this important preliminary, all "explanations" of evil and their refutations are reduced to the level of an odiously, ludicrously speculative massacre. But we can understand how arguments bear witness in their own way to a deeper intention which deserves to be read behind the explanation.

Finally, it is this intention, this testimony behind an explanation, that I endeavor to study in the last two chapters, by coming back in a personal way to what I called *"implications."*

"Testimony I" *recounts* a stage of the past, the validity of which I do not now entirely deny: The Promethean attitude, from its particular standpoint, has a degree of correctness and deserves to be understood. But there is more; this stage takes on a new meaning both by the continuity and discontinuity which tie it in with "Testimony II."

This trajectory seemed to me to be exemplary – as do all living evolutions. By no means is there ever a question in this subject of demonstrating anything. Everyone testifies in his own way and is incapable of totally putting himself in someone else's place. The important point is not always the opinion we have, but the road leading to that opinion. We are dealing with a history, a duration which we could not afford to do without; things are not true in the same way *before* and *after* that "narrow passage" (in speleological terms) which is only negotiated at the price of a hard squeeze. My goal was to describe the difficulties of and solutions for such a passage.

If the last chapter leads someone to believe that I have fallen into a more or less apologetical or moralizing viewpoint, back onto the old saw of "redeeming pain" after having criticized these saws to the very extent of my capabilities, it is only because I have poorly expressed myself. It is one thing to adopt a prepared set of morals and another to arrive at a practical knowledge (a "praxis," where judgment and action are united) while going to the end of a road consisting of bitter, negative, critical cleansing. Thus we understand the significance of certain shocking pages on evil which now belong to the past in which they were written but which I desired to situate as a moment in an evolution. After them, it is impossible to confuse "Testimony II" with some moralizing or pseudoreligious salvaging (or destruction) of pain!

Our plan throughout this book has been to follow this curve with its different stages and difficulties.

Thus warned, the reader can understand this *in another way:* It all may be summed up in a simple sentence, "We endow pain with meaning and with meaninglessness."

1. *We?* Following classical apologetics, evil is only an illusion of our limited view. A revolting explanation!

2. *We?* Following the revolted viewpoint of our former critical attitude, our pride would do away with evil by jealously keeping the pleasure of our having followed the path from ourselves to evil. This would be a proffered grace, not a received grace.

3. *We?* Following a viewpoint of received grace, evil becomes what our work makes of it, and we attain hope. This experience (of hope) describes my position today.

I have never been satisfied with the metaphysical explanations of evil: multiplicity, dispersion, individuality, falling back, stopping, descent, procession, separation, and fall in time.[1] All of this is *neutral.* Evil is more than a "distance," even an objectified distance; it designates a *refused* distance. Evil is only evil because of man's negation of a proffered gift—*that distance, which is then called exile.*[2]

No *objective* description of evil is possible. No description of matter and multiplicity, of time and dissolution, is sufficient if man does not admit the hidden presence of his *refusal.* In order for evil to exist, man must oppose a certain reality with his *no.* This *"no" is the other name for pain.*

Pain is our refusal, our *no,* the painful cry of man in revolt against a certain reality in his own flesh.

[1] We have already seen the ambivalence between the fall into individualism and multiplicity, and time. For although the dualistic, segregating time of the critical stage in man's evolution may designate the symbolic place of a fall into dispersion; on the other hand, the time which is that of creative duration, a part of continual maturation, of growth, of fulfillment, is significant as a redemption, a return from exile. Cf. Mme. Lévy-Valensi, *Les niveaux de l'etre* [The levels of being] (Paris: Presses Universitaires de France, 1962). Intuition transcends critical dualism and becomes one with the One, with creative time itself. Over against the time of evolution, of accomplishment (of the "end of time"), is the time of involution.

[2] The decisive baptism, as *exile,* of an objective distance (incorrectly called "metaphysical evil" since the time of Leibnitz) is our present concern, but it would deserve to be emphasized in the work I have just quoted (preceding note): the passage from an abstract metaphysics of evil as a "procession" to a concrete metaphysics of exile, a *refused* procession.

Excrement would be only a "fact of life," were it not for man's sense of smell which gives it a negative sign, makes it nauseating.

If man's *no* (whether justified or not is of little importance here) is the creator or co-creator of evil; his *yes,* on the other hand, wipes out evil and transforms pain. *Yes* is the key word to every form of asceticism (Hindu, Stoic, Christian also; it is acceptance, so different from resignation) : *yes* to my pain, to my aging, to my death, to a universal One, to God's will. This *yes* is called renouncement, availability, liberty, reconciliation with the world and with oneself. Every great wisdom movement has taught it. Instead of only wearing myself out trying to get the world to march in step with me, I must also do my part in regulating my steps to the rhythm of the universe. Technique must be married with asceticism.

No and *evil* interpenetrate; they are identical. This identity may be understood in three ways:

1. The *no* of revolt/sin is evil telescoped into moral evil.
2. The *no* of human consciousness in revolt at the sight of a suffering child is moral evil telescoped into suffered evil.
3. I see an intermediary *no,* as it were, a *no* which is a constituting element in the dualistic or critical moment in human evolution, divided within itself – a disproportionate being.

Without man's *no,* whatever the meanings that may be attributed to it, no reality deserves to be evil – death is no more serious than the erosion of the earth; a broken leg is no more or less than the eruption of a volcano or the typhoon which comes through and lays low an entire continent.

Going through and then beyond this intermediary *no,* the *yes* of hope and of work is an astonishing stubbornness, transforming the world before our very eyes.